NEUROLOGY - LABORATORY AND
RESEARCH DEVELOPMENTS

AUTOIMMUNITY TO NEURONAL PROTEINS IN NEUROLOGICAL DISORDERS

NEUROLOGY - LABORATORY AND CLINICAL RESEARCH DEVELOPMENTS

Additional books in this series can be found on Nova's website under the Series tab.

Additional E-books in this series can be found on Nova's website under the E-book tab.

NEUROLOGY - LABORATORY AND CLINICAL
RESEARCH DEVELOPMENTS

AUTOIMMUNITY TO NEURONAL PROTEINS IN NEUROLOGICAL DISORDERS

SANDRA AMOR

AND

RUTH HUIZINGA

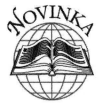

Nova Science Publishers, Inc.
New York

LIBRARY OF CONGRESS CATALOGING-IN-PUBLICATION DATA

Amor, Sandra.
  Autoimmunity to neuronal proteins in neurological disorders / authors, Sandra Amor, Ruth Huizinga.
    p. ; cm.
  Includes bibliographical references and index.
  ISBN 978-1-61324-397-8 (softcover)
  1. Nervous system--Diseases--Immunological aspects. 2. Autoimmune diseases. 3. Nerve tissue proteins. I. Huizinga, Ruth. II. Title.
  [DNLM: 1. Nervous System Diseases--immunology. 2. Autoimmunity. 3. Nerve Tissue Proteins--immunology. WL 140]
  RC346.5.A46 2011
  616.8'0479--dc22
                                                                    2011011459

Published by Nova Science Publishers, Inc. ✝ New York

CONTENTS

PREFACE

The brain is often referred to as being an immune-privilege site implying that trafficking of immune cells and molecules into the central nervous system (CNS) is limited or controlled so as to prevent collateral damage. Nevertheless, there is increasing evidence demonstrating complex interactions between the immune system and the nervous systems. Immune cells and their secreted substances – cytokine, chemokines and growth factors modulate the cells of the nervous system. Equally it is well know that events such as psychological stress impact on the immune system modulating its effect in the periphery. Glia cells also engaged in immunological reactions while immune and regulatory molecules expressed by neurons aid the control of otherwise damaging immune responses as well as encourage neuroprotective pathways. More recently studies show that complement aids the elimination of synapses while MHC class I molecules have a dramatic effect on the anatomy and physiology of neurological synapse.

One interaction between the immune system and nervous system that is more frequently observed is the generation of autoimmunity to neuronal antigens. Autoimmunity is involved in a diverse number of neurological disorders affecting both the central and peripheral nervous system. Commonly antibodies to neuronal antigens are observed in paraneoplastic disorders and although it is unclear what the exact role of the antibodies and indeed T cells are at least in some disorders their presence is linked with neurological disease. Autoantibodies to neuronal antigens are also observed in neurodegenerative disease, movement disorders, following infections and in chronic diseases such multiple sclerosis. In the latter disease the view that autoreactive T-cells directed to myelin proteins in the CNS are fundamental in the pathology of demyelinating disorders such as MS has dominated neuroimmunology research for many years. This has led to the reliance on experimental models of paralytic neurological disease, namely experimental autoimmune encephalomyelitis, induced in susceptible animals by immunisation of myelin proteins. However autoimmunity to neuronal antigens is also described in MS and thus may contribute to the axonal damage and neurodegeneration observed.

The increasing evidence for the role of autoimmunity to neuronal proteins in both peripheral and central nervous system disorders has led to the development of animal models and in vitro systems to probe the human disorders. Moreover, the recognition that autoimmunity to neuronal antigens is associated with a variety of neurological disorders has led to the implementation of immunotherapy. In this book the authors review the evidence for autoimmunity to neurons and axons in neurological diseases, discuss the animal models that are used to study the mechanisms of disease and indicate how such autoimmunity is relevant for therapies in these disorders.

In Chapter 1 the authors discuss how the CNS limits immune activation due to its immune privilege status. Nevertheless immune responses do take place in the CNS sometimes with devastating consequences. Neurons and other glia cells are damaged by activation of the innate and adaptive immune responses and autoimmunity to neuronal cells arise due to a number of different mechanisms. The Authors discuss this further in the following chapters. In Chapter 2 diseases of neuromuscular junction including myasthenia gravis - a model autoimmune disorder of the peripheral nervous system and other autoimmune disorders of the peripheral nervous system are discussed including disorders where antibodies are directed to the muscle-specific kinase and nerve terminal voltage-gated calcium channels. Other peripheral neuropathies, including Guillain-Barré syndrome as well as, diabetes in which autoimmunity to neuronal antigens is sometimes observed, are reviewed in Chapter 3. Chapter 4 covers the paraneoplastic disorders in which tumours trigger autoimmune responses in both the peripheral as well as the central nervous system. In Chapter 5 The Authors review movement disorders such as Sydenham's Chorea. The neurodegenerative diseases amyotrophic lateral sclerosis and Alzheimer's disease have distinct clinical manifestation yet both involve degeneration of neurons in which there is evidence for the involvement of innate and adaptive immune responses. In particular activated microglia are found at site of damage indicting innate immune activation. Yet the adaptive immune responses are also thought to be involved and these ideas are discussed in Chapter 6 while in Chapter 7 the authors discuss the role of autoimmunity to neuronal antigens in other disorders such as psychiatric disorders.

Chapter 8 covers multiple sclerosis thought to be an autoimmune disease in which autoimmune T and B cells responses, long thought to be directed to myelin, have more recently found to also be directed to neuronal antigens. In many of these chapters the authors have included animal models of those disorders which have helped dissect the pathogenic responses and highlighted the role of protective immune responses. In Chapter 9 the authors have reviewed the different mechanisms by which the autoimmune response may trigger neuronal damage. In the final Chapter 10 the authors review the therapies that are currently used for neurodegenerative disorders including amyotrophic lateral sclerosis and Alzheimer's disease, brain trauma, multiple sclerosis several of the paraneoplastic neurodegenerative disorders and Parkinson's disease. Theauthors first focus on those approaches that target the immune response in disorders in which the immune responses has been shown to play a key role in the disease such as myasthenia gravis, paraneoplastic disorders and multiple sclerosis. In the second part the neuroprotective approaches are discussed including existing approved compounds as well as experimental approaches to treat these disorders.

Chapter 1

NEURONS AND AXONS AS TARGET OF THE IMMUNE RESPONSE

Ruth Huizinga[1] and Sandra Amor[2,3]
[1] Department of Immunology, Erasmus MC,
University Medical Center, Rotterdam, The Netherlands.
[2] Department of Pathology, VU Medical Center Amsterdam,
The Netherlands.
[3] Neuroscience and Trauma Centre,
Barts and the London School of Medicine and Dentistry,
Queen Mary University of London, United Kingdom.

INTRODUCTION

Neuroimmunology is a rapidly developing area revealing the interactions between the immune system and the peripheral and central nervous systems. Despite such interactions in which the immune system is generally considered to be the detrimental partner, the CNS has developed strategies that aim to limit pathogenic immune responses in the CNS. This so-called phenomenon of "immune privilege" was recognized by Medawar early in the 19th century and has led to the idea that immune responses are tightly regulated in the CNS. Such regulation is in part dependent on the blood-brain barrier (BBB) designed to limit entry of solutes and ions (Figure 1) by means of the cellular components as well as molecular components such as the multidrug resistant proteins. Evidence for the existence of the BBB arose from the early studies by

Paul Ehrlich showing that peripheral injection of intravital dyes stained the organs and tissues while leaving the brain was unaffected. As well as the BBB endothelial cells, basement membranes and multidrug resistant proteins astrocytes and microglia also play a major role in the regulation of molecules and cells entering the CNS. It is often assumed that neurons play a passive role in immune regulation in the CNS and they are generally thought of as being the victims of unwanted immune responses. However neurons produce neuropeptides and transmitters that in addition to the neuronal membrane molecules all regulate inflammation (Amor *et al.*, 2010). Neurons express low levels of major histocompatibility complex (MHC) molecules while actively promoting T-cell apoptosis via the Fas-Fas ligand pathway (CD95-CD95L). While this approach is protective in health it is clear that damaged neurons are less able to maintain this protective shield allowing further insults.

Despite efforts to limit an otherwise damaging environment within the CNS, immune responses are clearly crucial to control neurotropic infections and for example restore homeostasis following ischemia. The key point is whether these immune responses also contribute to the neuronal damage in neurological disorders such as viral infection and chronic disorders such as multiple sclerosis.

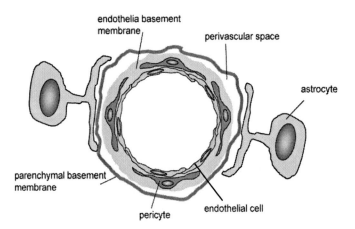

Figure 1. The blood brain barrier - BBB. Components of the BBB include the endothelial cells with specialised tight junctions, the endothelia basement membranes and the parenchyma basement membranes. In addition the end-feet of astrocytes are in close contact with the parenchymal basement membranes aiding the integrity of the BBB.

MULTIPLE SCLEROSIS – AN AUTOIMMUNE DISORDER?

Multiple sclerosis (MS) is a chronic inflammatory demyelinating disease in which autoreactive T-cell responses to myelin proteins in the central nervous system (CNS) are widely believed to contribute to the pathology. This view has dominated the research field in MS for many years and led to the reliance on experimental models of neurological disease following immunisation with myelin antigens. Such experimental diseases have developed as the central paradigm to investigate underlying mechanisms operating in MS as well as the preclinical development of therapeutic strategies. This long-standing concept has recently shifted and evidence is rapidly accumulating indicting a significance role of axonal damage and neurodegeneration in disease. Indeed axonal damage is now considered to be the major cause of irreversible neurological disability in MS patients. One correlate of axonal damage in MS is the presence of antibodies against neurofilament light protein, a major component of the axonal cytoskeleton. Contrary to extensive literature on pathogenic myelin autoimmunity the possible pathogenic role of autoimmunity to axonal antigens in MS has so far been ignored. Our recent experimental data indicate that autoimmunity to axonal antigens, as described in MS, is pathogenic rather than acting merely as a surrogate marker for axonal degeneration.

DEFINING CRITERIA FOR AUTOIMMUNE DISEASE

As validation of the concept that autoimmunity directed to neuronal antigens plays a role in disease we define four criteria – the so-called Witebsky's Criteria (Box 1). First that autoreactivity to neuronal antigens are consistently present in neurological disease in humans and experimental neurological disease in animals. Secondly that transfer of such neuronal reactive T cells and/or antibodies are pathogenic either *in vivo* or *in vitro* model systems. Thirdly, that immunization with neuronal antigens induces pathogenic autoimmune responses and leads to neurological disease in experimental animals and finally that inhibition of such responses ameliorates neurological disease.

Using these criteria we review the evidence for autoimmunity to neuronal antigens in several neurodegenerative disorders such as paraneoplastic disorders, and discuss how similar mechanisms may also operate in MS. Using the experimental models we describe our recent data to indicate that while clinical disease in MS models is due to autoimmune attack on myelin, neurons and axons can be also target for pathogenic autoimmunity. Understanding the factors leading to neuronal injury and neurodegenerative disorders is key to the development of effective therapies to prevent progression of disease and irreversible damage.

Circumstantial evidence
Autoantibodies and T cells to neuronal antigens
  a)   are present in patients with neurological disease
  b)   recognize neuronal and axonal targets

Direct Evidence
Autoantibodies and T cells to neuronal antigens
  a)   adoptively transfer disease in animals
  b)   immunization with the neuronal antigen induces the neurological disease in animals

Box 1. Witebsky's criteria.

IMMUNITY TO NEURONS AND AXONS

The immune responses must maximise the removal of harmful microorganisms while protecting the healthy tissues and cells. In the CNS this protection is exemplified in part by the presence of the blood brain barrier (BBB) and low level expression of molecules on neurons required for immune activation as well as expression of molecules crucial for tissue protection and repair.

To exert a pathogenic effect on neurons and axons T cells need to recognise antigenic peptides presented by the major histocompatibility complex (MHC) molecules. Antigens derived from endogenously synthesised proteins are bound to MHC class I molecules and are recognised by CD8 positive (CD8+) T cells whereas antigens derived from proteins, internalised by endocytosis and processed in vesicles, are bound to MHC class II molecules and recognised by CD4 positive (CD4+) T cells. However, in health the CNS and in particular neurons are protected in part from pathogenic immunity by the blood brain barrier but also by expression of low levels of MHC molecules. The situation is different in disease where the expression of MHC molecules is dependent in the type of tissue injury. In MS lesions neurons and axons express Class I but not MHC class II molecules (Hoftberger *et al.*, 2004, Neumann *et al.*, 1995) and thus may be target for Class I restricted killing. Indeed CD8+ cytotoxic T cell induced neuronal damage in dorsal root ganglia is a prominent feature in viral infections such as lentivirus infections (Zhu *et al.*, 2006) although the exact role of T cells in neurodegenerative disorders is unknown.

EVIDENCE FOR AUTOIMMUNITY TO AXONAL ANTIGENS

The precise role of pathogenic autoimmunity to self antigens including neuronal and myelin antigens, as has been described in several neuronal disorders although in all these cases is difficult to establish. The mere presence of antibodies and T cell responses to CNS antigens in human disease is clearly insufficient to assume that autoimmunity is relevant to disease or damage in the CNS. Firm evidence for the role of autoimmunity to axonal antigens in neurological disorders heavily relies on the pathogenic effect of autoreactive T cells and antibodies in cell culture and *in vivo* or following immunisation of experimental animals with neuronal proteins. Nevertheless many neuronal antigens and immune responses to neuronal antigens have been associated with human disorders (Table 1) in particular with the PND (see chapter 4).

To rationally examine the evidence for a pathogenic effect of autoimmunity to axonal antigens in neurological disorders we believe that the evidence should fulfil Witebsky's criteria (Rose and Bona, 1993) [Box 1]. These include *indirect* (circumstantial) evidence from clinical clues in patients i.e. a) the autoantibody or T cell should be present in the patient with disease; b) the autoantibody and/or T cells recognises the specific antigen, and *direct* evidence in which c) antibodies or T cells from patients are pathogenic to neuronal cells *in vitro* or induce neurological disease in laboratory animals and d) immunisation of the animal with the antigen should mimic the disease in humans.

Most of the direct evidence for a pathogenic role of anti-neuronal autoimmunity in humans comes from studying the effects of antibodies and T cells from patients with neurological disease *in vitro* on neuronal cell cultures. Adoptive transfer of T cells and antibodies *in vivo* has proven to be more difficult probably due to the difficulty in directing antibodies into the PNS or CNS due to the blood nerve barrier or BBB. Furthermore the pathogenic action of antibodies may rely on uptake by or entry into neurons via species specific pathways e.g. FcR receptors. In the case of FcR mouse Fc receptors are known to have different functions than those of humans and moreover the

Fc portion of human immunoglobulins may not be recognised by rodents FcR. Likewise, activated T cells from humans may not recognise antigen due to sequence differences or due to inadequate presentation by murine antigen presenting cells. Thus transferring immunoglobulin or T cells from patients to mice or other animals must be viewed with caution.

Many neurological disorders are associated with antibodies to neuronal antigens however in some case cellular responses are also observed. Evidence that T cells may be involved in the pathogenicity of neurodegenerative disorders comes from the observation of T cells in the nervous system as well as the CSF and blood both in the PNS and CNS disorders. T -cells are present in the spinal cord from patients with ALS, MS, GBS as well as patients with paraneoplastic cerebellar degeneration. In many cases it is unclear what these T cells recognise and indeed whether they are pathogenic.

ANIMAL MODELS

Despite their limitations animal models can be crucial tools in defining the pathogenesis of human diseases and are essential to develop and examine the safety of therapeutic interventions for patients with complex neuroimmunological syndromes. For example, the autoimmune basis of MS is well-accepted. This has been partly supported by the rodent and primate models which replicate many but not all of the pathological features (Amor *et al.*, 2005, Brok *et al.*, 2001). It is worth noting that animal models themselves must also be viewed with caution as being an analogue rather than the exact copy of the human counterpart, because they invariably differ to some degree from the human disease.

Due to the wide variety of biological tools available, rodent models are the most widely used system to probe the mechanisms underlying human disorders. Moreover, the extensive numbers of mutant mice deficient in specific immune factors allow detailed investigation of the disease models. These include mice deficient in FcR, B cells or TCR, or SCID mice which can be reconstituted to examine individual components of the immune response or indeed 'humanised' by reconstituting with human cells. For several neurodegenerative diseases models in non-human primates (Eslamboli, 2005) such as Parkinson's disease may be more relevant since behavioural studies such as cognitive changes can be better investigated in higher species (Philippens *et al.*, 2000).

Table 1. Distribution of neuronal antigens, immune responses and disease association

Antigens	Expression and role	Disease association with antineuronal antigens	Reference
Neurofilament-light	Axons – intracellular component Control of axonal calibre and axonal transport	ALS, Axonal neuropathy, MS	Couratier et al., 1998 Silber et al., 2002
Neurofilament-heavy	Axons - intracellular component Control of axonal calibre and axonal transport	Alzheimer's disease, GBS	Soussan et al., 1994 Terryberry et al., 1998
GluR3	Glutamate subunit on postsynaptic cell surface protein	Rasmussen's encephalitis	Levite and Hermelin 1999
aldolase C monomeric γ-gamma-enolase pyruvate kinase dimeric γ-enolase	40, 45, 60 and 98 kDa proteins of neurons	Basal ganglion disease, Encephalitis lethargica. Sydenham's Chorea Tourette's syndrome	Martino and Giovannoni 2004 Church et al., 2002 Church et al., 2003 Hallet et al., 2000
Tau	Microtubule-associated protein that stabilizes neuronal microtubules	Alzheimer's disease	Rosenman et al., 2006
NR2A and NR2B	Neurons in hippocampus, amygdale and hypothalamus Subunits of NMDA receptor	SLE	Huerta et al., 2006 Sakic 2005 DeGiorgio et al., 2001
Beta-III-tubulin	Neuronal cytoskeleton	Brain trauma, CIDP	Skoda et al., 2006
Gangliosides GM1; GQ1b GD1b GD1a GalNAc-GD1a	Cell membranes – enriched in neurons	ALS MFS; cerebellar ataxia Ataxic sensory neuropathy GD1a GalNAc-GD1a	Hughes and Cornblath 2005 Goodfellow et al., 2005
GAD	Synapses, nerve terminals GABAnergic neurons	Stiff person syndrome in association with diabetes	Schloot et al., 1999

Table 2. Neurological disease in animals immunised with neuronal antigens

Human disease	Animal strain	Immunisation/procedure	Reference
Myasthenia Gravis	mouse mouse rabbits rhesus monkeys	torpedo AChR in CFA MuSK extracellular domain MuSK extracellular domain torpedo AChR	Drachman et al., 1998 Christadoss et al., 2000 Jha et al., 2006 Shigemoto et al., 2006 Toro-Goyco et al., 1986
LEMS	rats mice	synaptotagmin peptides	Takamori et al., 1994
GBS	mice rabbits guinea pigs	lipooligosaccharide of B. melitensis ganglioside or galactocerebrosides C jujuni LOS	Watanabe et al., 2005 Caporale et al., 2006; Saida et al., 1981; Shu et al., 2006
Paraneoplastic neurodegenerative disorders e.g. HuD PNMA1 (Ma1)	mice rats	Immunization with plasmid coding HuD and implantation with neuroblastoma cell line Immunisation with, and transfer of Ma specific T cells	Carpentier et al., 1998 Pellkofer et al., 2004
SPS	rats	*Passive transfer SPS patients Ig to amphiphysin'	Sommer et al., 2005
Diabetes neuropathy	mice, rats	neuropathy in diabetic mice and following T cell transfer	Calcutt 2002; Schmidt et al., 2003; Bour-Jordan et al., 2005
Movement disorders Sydenhamn's Chorea Tourette's syndrome	SJL/J mice	Homogenate of group A beta-haemolytic streptococcal bacteria in CFA.	Hoffman et al., 2004
Amyotrophic lateral sclerosis	guinea pigs	bovine spinal motor neurons spinal cord ventral horn homogenate choline acetyltransferase	Engelhardt 1990

Alzheimer's disease	rats	cholinergic neurons.	Chapman et al., 1989
	rats	peptides of B-sunuclein	Mor et al., 2003
	mice	recombinant human tau protein	Rosenmann et al., 2006b.
	rats	cholinergic Torpedo neurons.	Michaelson et al., 1990
	rats	with NF-H protein of cholinergic neurons	Oron et al., 1997
	guinea pigs	with septal cholinergic neurons	Kalman et al., 1997
Parkinson's Disease	guinea pigs	homogenates of bovine mesencephalon dopaminergic MES 23.5 cells	Appel et al., 1992; Le et al., 1995
Brain Trauma	rats	brain trauma fluid percussion injury	Hoshino et al., 1996 Rudehill et al., 2006
Epilepsy; Rasmussen's syndrome	mice	Glu3RB peptide aa 372-395	Levite and Hermelin 1999
	rabbits	Glu3R fragment aa residues 245-457	Twyman et al., 1995
SLE	MRL/lpr mouse	spontaneous	Hikawa et al., 1997; Ballok et al., 2004; Sidor et al., 2005

AChR, acetylcholine receptors. CFA, complete Freund's adjuvant. *only passive transfer of antibodies.

Taking these factors into account in the following chapters we discuss the evidence for pathogenic responses of T cells and antibodies to neuronal antigens from patients with neurological disease *in vitro*. In addition, we will outline the major models of diseases in which autoimmunity to neuronal structures have been demonstrated (Table 2). These experimental models provide evidence that autoimmunity to neuronal antigens may contribute to the disease process rather than act as markers of neuronal damage, or are secondary to neuronal damage, or being an epiphenomenon.

REFERENCES

Amor S, Puentes F, Baker D, van der Valk P. 2010 Inflammation in neurodegenerative diseases *Immunology.* 129:154-69.

Amor S, Smith PA, Hart B and Baker D 2005. Biozzi mice: of mice and human neurological diseases. *J. Neuroimmunol.* 165: 1-10.

Appel SH, Le WD, Tajti J, Haverkamp LJ and Engelhardt JI 1992. Nigral damage and dopaminergic hypofunction in mesencephalon-immunized guinea pigs. *Ann. Neurol.* 32: 494-501.

Ballok DA, Earls AM, Krasnik C, Hoffman SA and Sakic B 2004. Autoimmune-induced damage of the midbrain dopaminergic system in lupus-prone mice. *J. Neuroimmunol.* 152: 83-97.

Bour-Jordan H, Thompson HL and Bluestone JA 2005. Distinct effector mechanisms in the development of autoimmune neuropathy versus diabetes in nonobese diabetic mice. *J. Immunol.* 175: 5649-55.Brok HP, Bauer J, Jonker M, Blezer E, Amor S, Bontrop RE, Laman JD and t Hart BA 2001. Non-human primate models of multiple sclerosis. *Immunol. Rev.* 183: 173-85.

Calcutt NA 2002. Future treatments for diabetic neuropathy: clues from experimental neuropathy. *Curr. Diab. Rep.* 2: 482-8.

Caporale CM, Capasso M, Luciani M, Prencipe V, Creati B, Gandolfi P, De Angelis MV, Di Muzio A, Caporale V and Uncini A 2006. Experimental axonopathy induced by immunization with Campylobacter jejuni lipopolysaccharide from a patient with Guillain-Barre syndrome. *J. Neuroimmunol.* 174: 12-20.

Carpentier AF, Rosenfeld MR, Delattre JY, Whalen RG, Posner JB and Dalmau J 1998. DNA vaccination with HuD inhibits growth of a neuroblastoma in mice. *Clin. Cancer Res.* 4: 2819-24.

Chapman J, Feldon J, Alroy G and Michaelson DM 1989. Immunization of rats with cholinergic neurons induces behavioral deficits. *J. Neural. Transplant.* 1: 63-76.

Church AJ, Cardoso F, Dale RC, Lees AJ, Thompson EJ and Giovannoni G 2002. Anti-basal ganglia antibodies in acute and persistent Sydenham's chorea. *Neurology.* 59: 227-31.

Church AJ, Dale RC, Cardoso F, Candler PM, Chapman MD, Allen ML, Klein NJ, Lees AJ and Giovannoni G 2003. CSF and serum immune parameters in Sydenham's chorea: evidence of an autoimmune syndrome? *J. Neuroimmunol.* 136: 149-53.

Christadoss P, Poussin M and Deng C 2000. Animal models of myasthenia gravis. *Clin. Immunol.* 94: 75-87.

Couratier P, Yi FH, Preud'homme JL, Clavelou P, White A, Sindou P, Vallat JM and Jauberteau MO 1998. Serum autoantibodies to neurofilament proteins in sporadic amyotrophic lateral sclerosis. *J. Neurol. Sci.* 154: 137-45.

DeGiorgio LA, Konstantinov KN, Lee SC, Hardin JA, Volpe BT and Diamond B 2001. A subset of lupus anti-DNA antibodies cross-reacts with the NR2 glutamate receptor in systemic lupus erythematosus. *Nat. Med.* 7: 1189-93.

Drachman DB, McIntosh KR and Yang B 1998. Factors that determine the severity of experimental myasthenia gravis. *Ann. N. Y. Acad. Sci.* 841: 262-82.

Engelhardt JI, Appel SH and Killian JM 1990. Motor neuron destruction in guinea pigs immunized with bovine spinal cord ventral horn homogenate: experimental autoimmune gray matter disease. *J. Neuroimmunol.* 27: 21-31.

Eikelenboom MJ, Petzold A, Lazeron RH, Silber E, Sharief M, Thompson EJ, Barkhof F, Giovannoni G, Polman CH and Uitdehaag BM 2003. Multiple sclerosis: Neurofilament light chain antibodies are correlated to cerebral atrophy. *Neurology.* 60: 219-23.

Eslamboli A 2005. Marmoset monkey models of Parkinson's disease: which model, when and why? *Brain Res. Bull.* 68: 140-9.

Goodfellow JA, Bowes T, Sheikh K, Odaka M, Halstead SK, Humphreys PD, Wagner ER, Yuki N, Furukawa K, Plomp JJ and Willison HJ 2005. Overexpression of GD1a ganglioside sensitizes motor nerve terminals to anti-GD1a antibody-mediated injury in a model of acute motor axonal neuropathy. *J. Neurosci.* 25: 1620-8.

Hallett JJ, Harling-Berg CJ, Knopf PM, Stopa EG and Kiessling LS 2000. Anti-striatal antibodies in Tourette syndrome cause neuronal dysfunction. *J. Neuroimmunol.* 111: 195-202.

Hikawa N, Kiuchi Y, Maruyama T and Takenaka T 1997. Delayed neurite regeneration and its improvement by nerve growth factor (NGF) in dorsal root ganglia from MRL-lpr/lpr mice in vitro. *J. Neurol. Sci.* 149: 13-7.

Hoftberger R, Aboul-Enein F, Brueck W, Lucchinetti C, Rodriguez M, Schmidbauer M, Jellinger K and Lassmann H 2004. Expression of major histocompatibility complex class I molecules on the different cell types in multiple sclerosis lesions. *Brain Pathol.* 14: 43-50.

Huerta PT, Kowal C, DeGiorgio LA, Volpe BT and Diamond B 2006. Immunity and behavior: antibodies alter emotion. *Proc. Natl. Acad. Sci. U. S. A.* 103: 678-83.

Hughes RA and Cornblath DR 2005. Guillain-Barre syndrome. *Lancet.* 366: 1653-66.

Hoffman KL, Hornig M, Yaddanapudi K, Jabado O and Lipkin WI 2004. A murine model for neuropsychiatric disorders associated with group A beta-hemolytic streptococcal infection. *J. Neurosci.* 24: 1780-91.

Hoshino S, Kobayashi S and Nakazawa S 1996. Prolonged and extensive IgG immunoreactivity after severe fluid-percussion injury in rat brain. *Brain. Res* 711: 73-83.

Jha S, Xu K, Maruta T, Oshima M, Mosier DR, Atassi MZ and Hoch W 2006. Myasthenia gravis induced in mice by immunization with the recombinant extracellular domain of rat muscle-specific kinase (MuSK). *J. Neuroimmunol.* 175: 107-17.

Kalman J, Engelhardt JI, Le WD, Xie W, Kovacs I, Kasa P and Appel SH 1997. Experimental immune-mediated damage of septal cholinergic neurons. *J. Neuroimmunol.* 77: 63-74.

Le WD, Engelhardt J, Xie WJ, Schneider L, Smith RG and Appel SH 1995. Experimental autoimmune nigral damage in guinea pigs. *J. Neuroimmunol.* 57: 45-53.

Levite M and Hermelin A 1999. Autoimmunity to the glutamate receptor in mice--a model for Rasmussen's encephalitis? *J. Autoimmun.* 13: 73-82

Martino D and Giovannoni G 2004. Antibasal ganglia antibodies and their relevance to movement disorders. *Curr. Opin. Neurol.* 17: 425-32

Michaelson DM, Kadar T, Weiss Z, Chapman J and Feldon J 1990. Immunization with cholinergic cell bodies induces histopathological changes in rat brains. *Mol. Chem. Neuropathol.* 13: 71-80.

Mor F, Quintana F, Mimran A and Cohen IR 2003. Autoimmune encephalomyelitis and uveitis induced by T cell immunity to self beta-synuclein. *J. Immunol.* 170: 628-34.

Neumann H, Cavalie A, Jenne DE and Wekerle H 1995. Induction of MHC class I genes in neurons. *Science.* 269: 549-52.

Oron L, Dubovik V, Novitsky L, Eilam D and Michaelson DM 1997. Animal model and in vitro studies of anti neurofilament antibodies mediated neurodegeneration in Alzheimer's disease. *J. Neural Transm. Suppl.* 49: 77-84.

Pellkofer H, Schubart AS, Hoftberger R, Schutze N, Pagany M, Schuller M, Lassmann H, Hohlfeld R, Voltz R and Linington C 2004. Modelling paraneoplastic CNS disease: T-cells specific for the onconeuronal antigen PNMA1 mediate autoimmune encephalomyelitis in the rat. *Brain.* 127: 1822-30.

Philippens IH, Melchers BP, Roeling TA and Bruijnzeel PL 2000. Behavioral test systems in marmoset monkeys. *Behav. Res. Methods Instrum. Comput.* 32: 173-9.

Rose NR and Bona C 1993. Defining criteria for autoimmune diseases (Witebsky's postulates revisited). *Immunol. Today.* 14: 426-30.

Rosenmann H, Grigoriadis N, Karussis D, Boimel M, Touloumi O, Ovadia H and Abramsky O 2006a. Tauopathy-like abnormalities and neurologic deficits in mice immunized with neuronal tau protein. *Arch. Neurol.* 63: 1459-67.

Rudehill S, Muhallab S, Wennersten A, von Gertten C, Al Nimer F, Sandberg-Nordqvist AC, Holmin S and Mathiesen T 2006. Autoreactive antibodies against neurons and basal lamina found in serum following experimental brain contusion in rats. *Acta Neurochir. (Wien)* 148: 199-205; discussion 205.

Saida T, Saida K, Silberberg DH and Brown MJ 1981. Experimental allergic neuritis induced by galactocerebroside. *Ann. Neurol.* 9 Suppl: 87-101.

Sakic B, Kirkham DL, Ballok DA, Mwanjewe J, Fearon IM, Macri J, Yu G, Sidor MM, Denburg JA, Szechtman H, Lau J, Ball AK and Doering LC 2005. Proliferating brain cells are a target of neurotoxic CSF in systemic autoimmune disease. *J. Neuroimmunol.* 169: 68-85.

Schloot NC, Batstra MC, Duinkerken G, De Vries RR, Dyrberg T, Chaudhuri A, Behan PO and Roep BO 1999. GAD65-Reactive T cells in a non-diabetic stiff-man syndrome patient. *J. Autoimmun.* 12: 289-96.

Schmidt RE, Dorsey DA, Beaudet LN and Peterson RG 2003. Analysis of the Zucker Diabetic Fatty (ZDF) type 2 diabetic rat model suggests a neurotrophic role for insulin/IGF-I in diabetic autonomic neuropathy. *Am. J. Pathol.* 163: 21-8.

Shigemoto K, Kubo S, Maruyama N, Hato N, Yamada H, Jie C, Kobayashi N, Mominoki K, Abe Y, Ueda N and Matsuda S 2006. Induction of myasthenia by immunization against muscle-specific kinase. *J. Clin. Invest.* 116: 1016-24.

Shu XM, Cai FC and Zhang XP 2006. Carbohydrate mimicry of Campylobacter jejuni lipooligosaccharide is critical for the induction of anti-GM1 antibody and neuropathy. *Muscle Nerve.* 33: 225-31.

Sidor MM, Sakic B, Malinowski PM, Ballok DA, Oleschuk CJ and Macri J 2005. Elevated immunoglobulin levels in the cerebrospinal fluid from lupus-prone mice. *J. Neuroimmunol.* 165: 104-13.

Silber E, Semra YK, Gregson NA, Sharief MK. Patients with progressive multiple sclerosis have elevated antibodies to neurofilament subunit. *Neurology.* 2002 58:1372-81.

Skoda D, Kranda K, Bojar M, Glosova L, Baurle J, Kenney J, Romportl D, Pelichovska M and Cvachovec K 2006. Antibody formation against beta-tubulin class III in response to brain trauma. *Brain Res. Bull.* 68: 213-6.

Sommer C, Weishaupt A, Brinkhoff J, Biko L, Wessig C, Gold R and Toyka KV 2005. Paraneoplastic stiff-person syndrome: passive transfer to rats by means of IgG antibodies to amphiphysin. *Lancet.* 365: 1406-11Terryberry JW, Thor G and Peter JB 1998. Autoantibodies in neurodegenerative diseases: antigen-specific frequencies and intrathecal analysis. *Neurobiol. Aging.* 19: 205-16.

Soussan L, Tchernakov K, Bachar-Lavi O, Yuvan T, Wertman E and Michaelson DM 1994. Antibodies to different isoforms of the heavy neurofilament protein (NF-H) in normal aging and Alzheimer's disease. *Mol. Neurobiol.* 9: 83-91.

't Hart BA, Bauer J, Brok HP, Amor S. Non-human *J. Neuroimmunol.* 2005 Nov;168(1-2):1-12. Epub 2005 Jul 14.

Takamori M, Hamada T, Komai K, Takahashi M and Yoshida A 1994. Synaptotagmin can cause an immune-mediated model of Lambert-Eaton myasthenic syndrome in rats. *Ann. Neurol.* 35: 74-80.

Toro-Goyco E, Cora EM, Kessler MJ and Martinez-Carrion M 1986. Induction of experimental myasthenia gravis in rhesus monkeys: a model for the study of the human disease. *P. R. Health Sci. J.* 5: 13-8.

Trapp BD, Peterson J, Ransohoff RM, Rudick R, Mork S and Bo L 1998. Axonal transection in the lesions of multiple sclerosis. *N. Engl. J. Med.* 338: 278-85.

Twyman RE, Gahring LC, Spiess J and Rogers SW 1995. Glutamate receptor antibodies activate a subset of receptors and reveal an agonist binding site. *Neuron.* 14: 755-62.

Twyman RE, Gahring LC, Spiess J and Rogers SW 1995. Glutamate receptor antibodies activate a subset of receptors and reveal an agonist binding site. *Neuron.* 14: 755-62.

Watanabe K, Kim S, Nishiguchi M, Suzuki H and Watarai M 2005. Brucella melitensis infection associated with Guillain-Barre syndrome through molecular mimicry of host structures. *FEMS Immunol. Med. Microbiol.* 45: 121-7.

Zhu Y, Antony J, Liu S, Martinez JA, Giuliani F, Zochodne D and Power C 2006. CD8+ lymphocyte-mediated injury of dorsal root ganglion neurons during lentivirus infection: CD154-dependent cell contact neurotoxicity. *J. Neurosci.* 26: 3396-403.

Chapter 2

DISORDERS OF THE NEUROMUSCULAR JUNCTION

Ruth Huizinga[1] and Sandra Amor[2,3]

[1] Department of Immunology, Erasmus MC,
University Medical Center, Rotterdam, The Netherlands.
[2] Department of Pathology, VU Medical Center Amsterdam,
The Netherlands.
[3] Neuroscience and Trauma Centre,
Barts and the London School of Medicine and Dentistry,
Queen Mary University of London, United Kingdom.

INTRODUCTION

The neuromuscular junction allows transmission from the terminal of a motor neuron to the motor end plate of the muscle critical for muscle contraction. In myasthenia gravis - a model autoimmune disorder of the peripheral nervous system - autoantibodies to the muscle nicotinic acetylcholine receptor (AChR) on the post-synaptic endplate of the neuromuscular junction inhibit such transmission leading to muscle weakness. Autoantibodies to AChR are present in over 85% patients. Studies show that these antibodies are pathogenic in animals and induce muscle weakness similar to the human disease while therapies removing the antibodies are beneficial thereby fulfilling the Witebsky's criteria (see Chapter 1). As well as myasthenia gravis other autoimmune disorders of the peripheral nervous system are also well recognized in which antibodies recognize the muscle-specific kinase (MuSK) and nerve terminal voltage-gated calcium channels (VGCCs).

MYASTHENIA GRAVIS

Autoimmunity to antigens of the neuromuscular junction is observed in several neurological disorders such as the well-known disorder myasthenia gravis (MG) in which antibodies to acetylcholine receptor (AChR), an important neurotransmitter receptor results in weakness and fatigue (Vincent *et al.*, 1999; Vincent, 2006,). In many cases MG is associated with thymomas and therefore considered to belong to the group of diseases known as paraneoplastic disorders (see chapter 4). That antibodies to AChR may be pathogenic comes from indirect evidence in patients. Anti-AChR antibodies are observed in over 85% of MG patients where increasing levels of autoantibody correlate with deterioration in disease. In addition, MG patients respond to intravenous immunoglobulin (IvIg) which is thought to block the pathogenic antibodies. In mothers with MG anti-AChR antibodies cross the placenta or via the mother's milk enter the baby resulting in antibody-mediated *arthrogryposis multiplex congenita* (AMC) providing more direct evidence of autoimmunity in disease. However firm evidence for a pathogenic role of autoantibodies was first observed following passive transfer of serum from MG patients to mice (Toyka *et al.*, 1975). Following injection of the serum, mice developed neuromuscular defects associated with a reduction in the numbers of ACh receptors. In a follow up study the active fraction in the serum was identified as IgG and the effect was enhanced by complement component C3 (Toyka *et al.*, 1977). To address the role of autoreactive T cells in MG, lymphocytes from MG patients were transferred to SCID mice. In this study lymphocytes, activated to AChR epitopes, were purified to contain either CD4+ or CD8+ T cells. These studies clearly demonstrate that CD4+ T cells are crucial for the induction of experimental MG by providing 'help' to B cells in the production of pathogenic anti-AChR antibodies (Wang *et al.*, 1999).

As well as autoimmunity to AChR, MG is also associated with muscle atrophy in which antibodies to the muscle-specific kinase (MuSK) are observed (Hoch *et al.*, 2001). MuSK-related MG is clinically different from from AChR-related MG by the more frequent involvement of bulbar and cranial muscles. In addition, while in AChR-related MG IgG1 and

IgG3 AChR-reactive antibodies are found, MuSK-reactive antibodies are predominantly of the IgG4 isotype (McConville *et al.*, 2004).

Muscle biopsies from a patient with MuSK-specific antibodies showed electrophysiological abnormalities consistent with post-synaptic defects, while electron microscopy showed both pre- and post-synaptic degenerative changes (Niks *et al.*, 2010). Injection of MusK-specific antibodies isolated from MG patients into mice resulted in reduced expression of post-synaptic MuSK due to antibody-mediated internalisation (Cole *et al*, 2010). After one week of injections (45 μg / mouse / day), animals developed weight loss and muscle weakness, indicating that exposure to MuSK-specific antibodies induces clinical disease (Cole *et al.*, 2008).

AUTOIMMUNITY TO ION CHANNELS

Antibodies to ligand- and voltage-gated ion channels have been associated with a variety of clinical disorders in which defects in neuronal signalling and synaptic transmission are observed (Vincent, 2006). Lambert-Eaton myasthenic syndrome (LEMS) is a disorder frequently associated with small-cell lung cancer and is therefore considered a paraneoplastic disorder (see also chapter 4). LEMS can be clinically discriminated from MG by the presence of proximal limb weakness and more frequent autonomic dysfunction (Verschuuren *et al.*, 2010). The autoantibodies recognise voltage-gated calcium channels (VGCC) of the P/Q type, which are expressed pre-synaptically in neuromuscular junctions of skeletal muscle, the cerebellum and in the autonomic nervous system. The channels mediate Ca^{2+}-influx promoting exocytosis of ACh-containing vesicles. Antibodies to VGCC have been shown to decrease calcium currents in VGCC-transfected HEK293 cells (Lang and Vincent, 2003) and in rat Purkinje and granule cells, which express high levels of P/Q-type VGCC (Pinto *et al.*, 1998). In mice, VGCC-specific antibodies reduced the expression of calcium channels at the NMJ (Lang *et al.*, 2003).

Neuromyotonia, also known as Isaacs' syndrome, is another disorder of the PNS in which patients experience spontaneous muscle activity due to nerve hyperexcitability. The disease has been associated with antibodies to voltage-gated potassium channels (VGKC) (Shillito *et al.*, 1995). However, it became recently clear that the majority of VGKC-reactive antibodies do not recognise the ion channel itself but instead proteins that form complexes with VGKC, such as leucin-rich glioma inactivated-1 protein (Lgi1) or contactin-associated protein-2 (Caspr-2) (Irani *et al.*, 2010). While the pathogenic significance of these new autoantibodies has not been proven, earlier studies with VGKC-reactive F(ab')$_2$ fragments from neuromyotonia patients showed a decrease in VGKC expression and reduced potassium currents in neuroblastoma cells (Tomimitsu *et al.*, 2004). Antibodies to VGKC-associated proteins have also been described in disorders of the CNS such as limbic encephalitis and in patients with Morvan's syndrome, which have in addition to neuromyotonia also autonomic and CNS symptoms (Irani *et al.*, 2010, Lai *et al.*, 2010).

ANIMAL MODELS OF NEUROMUSCULAR AUTOIMMUNITY

Experimental autoimmune myasthenia gravis (EAMG) can be induced in many rodents by immunization with AChR from *Torpedo california* neurons or mouse AChR in complete Freund's adjuvant (Christadoss *et al.*, 2000). As with many models in mice (Drachman *et al.*, 1998) the MHC class II genes influence autoimmunity to AChR since MHC class II-restricted CD4+ cells are crucial for induction of anti-AChR antibodies. Moreover tolerance to AChR or dominant peptide epitopes prevents EAMG by blocking the action of these pathogenic T cells.

EAMG may also be induced following immunization of H-2(a), H-2(b), H-2(bm12) and H-2(d) mice with recombinant rat-MuSK extracellular domain (Jha *et al.*, 2006) although variations in clinical signs are observed. In rabbits immunization with the MuSK ectodomain protein induces MG-like muscle weakness with a reduction of AChR clustering at the NMJs (Shigemoto *et al.*, 2006) which more closely mimics the human disease.

Experimental models in higher species have also been developed, which are crucial for development of novel therapies as well as the study of effects of the disease on higher functions not possible in rodents. EAMG in rhesus monkeys may be induced with purified AChR from *Torpedo california* (Toro-Goyco *et al.*, 1986). Rhesus monkeys immunised with three doses of 80 mg protein at two-week intervals developed antibodies and clinical signs of disease correlating with the levels of antibodies induced. Histological examination revealed muscular atrophy, fibrous degeneration and lymphocyte infiltration in the lesions characteristic of MG.

In summary, MG serves as the prototypic disease fulfilling many criteria demonstrating a role for autoimmunity to neuronal antigens in disease. Not only do antibodies to MG correlate with disease but *in utero* transfer of antibodies in MG patients and transfer of human antibodies to AChR to animals mimics MG in humans. Evidence is also observed following immunisation of animals with purified AChR thus fulfilling Witebsky's criteria for pathogenic autoimmunity to axonal antigens in MG.

In LEMS the pathogenic role for antibodies to nerve terminal voltage-gated calcium channels (VGCCs) has been demonstrated in animals following chronic administration of plasma, serum or immunoglobulin G to mice. Following transfer, electrophysiological and ultrastructural findings similar to those seen in patients are observed (Flink and Atchison, 2003). These studies also showed a reduction in amplitude of Ca2+ currents through P/Q-type channels. In addition, transfer of antibodies to the presynaptic VGKC, the autoantigen in neuromyotonia, into mice also results in defects in neuromuscular transmission.

Immunisation with peptides of synaptotagmin, one of the functionally VGCC-associated proteins, induced electrophysiological changes following repeated injections of Lewis rats (Takamori et al., 1994). Whether active immunization with VGKC or associated proteins in experimental animals will mimic channelopathies in humans is unknown.

REFERENCES

Christadoss P, Poussin M and Deng C 2000. Animal models of myasthenia gravis. *Clin. Immunol.* 94: 75-87.

Cole RN, Ghazanfari N, Ngo ST, Gervasio OL, Reddel SW and Phillips WD 2010. Patient autoantibodies deplete postsynaptic muscle-specific kinase leading to disassembly of the ACh receptor scaffold and myasthenia gravis in mice. *J. Physiol.* 588: 3217-29.

Cole RN, Reddel SW, Gervasio OL and Phillips WD 2008. Anti-MuSK patient antibodies disrupt the mouse neuromuscular junction. *Ann. Neurol.* 63: 782-9.

Drachman DB, McIntosh KR and Yang B 1998. Factors that determine the severity of experimental myasthenia gravis. *Ann. N. Y. Acad. Sci.* 841: 262-82.

Flink MT and Atchison WD 2003. Ca2+ channels as targets of neurological disease: Lambert-Eaton Syndrome and other Ca2+ channelopathies. *J. Bioenerg. Biomembr.* 35: 697-718.

Hoch W, McConville J, Helms S, Newsom-Davis J, Melms A and Vincent A 2001. Auto-antibodies to the receptor tyrosine kinase MuSK in patients with myasthenia gravis without acetylcholine receptor antibodies. *Nat. Med.* 7: 365-8.

Irani SR, Alexander S, Waters P, Kleopa KA, Pettingill P, Zuliani L, Peles E, Buckley C, Lang B and Vincent A 2010. Antibodies to Kv1 potassium channel-complex proteins leucine-rich, glioma inactivated 1 protein and contactin-associated protein-2 in limbic encephalitis, Morvan's syndrome and acquired neuromyotonia. *Brain.* 133: 2734-48.

Jha S, Xu K, Maruta T, Oshima M, Mosier DR, Atassi MZ and Hoch W 2006. Myasthenia gravis induced in mice by immunization with the recombinant extracellular domain of rat muscle-specific kinase (MuSK). *J. Neuroimmunol.* 175: 107-17.

Lai M, Huijbers MG, Lancaster E, Graus F, Bataller L, Balice-Gordon R, Cowell JK and Dalmau J 2010. Investigation of LGI1 as the antigen in limbic encephalitis previously attributed to potassium channels: a case series. *Lancet Neurol.* 9: 776-85.

Lang B, Pinto A, Giovannini F, Newsom-Davis J and Vincent A 2003. Pathogenic autoantibodies in the Lambert Eaton myasthenic syndrome. *Ann. N. Y. Acad. Sci.* 998: 187-95.

Lang B and Vincent A 2003. Autoantibodies to ion channels at the neuromuscular junction. *Autoimmun. Rev.* 2: 94-100.

McConville J, Farrugia ME, Beeson D, Kishore U, Metcalfe R, Newsom-Davis J and Vincent A 2004. Detection and characterization of MuSK antibodies in seronegative myasthenia gravis. *Ann. Neurol.* 55: 580-4.

Niks EH, Kuks JB, Wokke JH, Veldman H, Bakker E, Verschuuren JJ and Plomp JJ 2010. Pre- and postsynaptic neuromuscular junction abnormalities in musk myasthenia. *Muscle Nerve.* 42: 283-8.

Pinto A, Gillard S, Moss F, Whyte K, Brust P, Williams M, Stauderman K, Harpold M, Lang B, Newsom-Davis J, Bleakman D, Lodge D and Boot J 1998. Human autoantibodies specific for the alpha1A calcium channel subunit reduce both P-type and Q-type calcium currents in cerebellar neurons. *Proc. Natl. Acad. Sci. U. S. A.* 95: 8328-33.

Shigemoto K, Kubo S, Maruyama N, Hato N, Yamada H, Jie C, Kobayashi N, Mominoki K, Abe Y, Ueda N and Matsuda S 2006. Induction of myasthenia by immunization against muscle-specific kinase. *J. Clin. Invest.* 116: 1016-24.

Shillito P, Molenaar PC, Vincent A, Leys K, Zheng W, van den Berg RJ, Plomp JJ, van Kempen GT, Chauplannaz G, Wintzen AR and et al. 1995. Acquired neuromyotonia: evidence for autoantibodies directed against K+ channels of peripheral nerves. *Ann. Neurol.* 38: 714-22.

Takamori M, Hamada T, Komai K, Takahashi M and Yoshida A 1994. Synaptotagmin can cause an immune-mediated model of Lambert-Eaton myasthenic syndrome in rats. *Ann. Neurol.* 35: 74-80.

Tomimitsu H, Arimura K, Nagado T, Watanabe O, Otsuka R, Kurono A, Sonoda Y, Osame M and Kameyama M 2004. Mechanism of action of voltage-gated K+ channel antibodies in acquired neuromyotonia. *Ann. Neurol.* 56: 440-4.

Toro-Goyco E, Cora EM, Kessler MJ and Martinez-Carrion M 1986. Induction of experimental myasthenia gravis in rhesus monkeys: a model for the study of the human disease. *P. R. Health Sci. J.* 5: 13-8.

Toyka KV, Brachman DB, Pestronk A and Kao I 1975. Myasthenia gravis: passive transfer from man to mouse. *Science.* 190: 397-9.

Toyka KV, Drachman DB, Griffin DE, Pestronk A, Winkelstein JA, Fishbeck KH and Kao I 1977. Myasthenia gravis. Study of humoral immune mechanisms by passive transfer to mice. *N. Engl. J. Med.* 296: 125-31.

Verschuuren JJ, Palace J and Gilhus NE 2010. Clinical aspects of myasthenia explained. *Autoimmunity.* 43: 344-52.

Vincent A 2006. Immunology of disorders of neuromuscular transmission. *Acta Neurol. Scand. Suppl.* 183: 1-7.

Vincent A, Lily O and Palace J 1999. Pathogenic autoantibodies to neuronal proteins in neurological disorders. *J. Neuroimmunol.* 100: 169-80.

Wang ZY, Karachunski PI, Howard JF, Jr. and Conti-Fine BM 1999. Myasthenia in SCID mice grafted with myasthenic patient lymphocytes: role of CD4+ and CD8+ cells. *Neurology.* 52: 484-97.

Chapter 3

IMMUNE-MEDIATED PERIPHERAL NEUROPATHIES

Ruth Huizinga[1] and Sandra Amor[2,3]

[1] Department of Immunology, Erasmus MC, University Medical Center, Rotterdam, The Netherlands.
[2] Department of Pathology, VU Medical Center Amsterdam, The Netherlands.
[3] Neuroscience and Trauma Centre, Barts and the London School of Medicine and Dentistry, Queen Mary University of London, United Kingdom.

INTRODUCTION

Autoimmunity to neuronal and axonal antigens has been reported in a variety of immune-mediated peripheral neuropathies, including acute diseases such as Guillain-Barré syndrome (GBS). In GBS, serum antibodies are predominantly directed to gangliosides, glycolipids that are highly enriched in the nervous system. These gangliosides antibodies are generated as a result of infection and cross-react with glycolipids. The neurotoxic potential of these antibodies has been demonstrated using *in vitro* culture systems and *in vivo* animal models. In human disorders peripheral neuropathy is also associated with chronic autoimmune diseases, for example diabetes and is associated with autoimmunity to axonal antigens. Here we review the evidence for autoimmunity to neuronal antigens in peripheral neuropathies and discuss the animal models of these disorders.

GUILLAIN-BARRÉ SYNDROME

GBS is a monophasic disorder associated with inflammation and nerve damage of the peripheral nervous system. GBS and related syndromes, such as Miller-Fisher syndrome (MFS) are strongly associated with bacterial and viral infections and are caused by antibody responses to gangliosides such as GM1 and GQ1b (Table 1). In approximately 25% of patients with GBS, particularly the axonal form, disease occurs after infection with *Campylobacter jejuni* which contains ganglioside-like structures similar to those of peripheral nerves. It has therefore been suggested that GBS is induced via the mechanism of molecular mimicry i.e. similarities between infectious agents and self antigens. Other infections that have also been associated with GBS include *Haemophilus influenzae*, *Mycoplasma pneumoniae*, Epstein-Barr virus and cytomegalovirus (Jacobs *et al.*, 1998). In these cases it is still unclear how these infections agents contribute to the disease process.

Table 1. Antibodies to gangliosides are associated with specific clinical diseases

Ganglioside	Disease	Expression	Reference
GM1, GM1b, GD1a, GalNAc-GD1a	Guillain-Barré syndrome	Motor nerve axons	(Gong *et al.*, 2002)
GD1b	Sensory ataxic neuropathy	Neurons of dorsal root ganglia	(Susuki *et al.*, 2001)
GQ1b	Miller-Fisher syndrome	Extraocular nerve terminals and muscle spindles	(Liu *et al.*, 2009)
GT1a	GBS with bulbar palsy	Lower cranial nerves	(Koga *et al.*, 2002)

Recently, it became clear that antibodies of some patients with GBS recognise glycolipid epitopes generated by different ganglioside molecules 'in complex'. For example the complex of GM1a with GD1b creates a novel epitope recognised by the serum of GBS patients but which do not show reactivity to the individual gangliosides (Kaida *et al.*, 2004). Importantly, the presence of ganglioside complexes can also prevent the binding and pathogenic activity of ganglioside-monoreactive antibodies, possibly explaining the heterogenic distribution of clinical symptoms in patients (Greenshields *et al.*, 2009).

In some patients with GBS, antibodies to neuronal antigens may also involve the CNS. For example, serum antibodies to GD1b and GM1 were elevated in a patient with GBS presenting with cerebellar ataxia (Bae and Kim, 2005). Further evidence is observed in Bickerstaff's encephalitis, a rare condition related to MFS involving the CNS in which antibodies to GQ1b gangliosides are thought to play a pathogenic role.

The pathogenicity of antibodies to gangliosides in GBS is proven by studies whereby transfer of serum and immunoglobulin from GBS patients induces neurodegenerative changes *in vivo* and physiological and pathological effects in culture. For example GBS sera containing anti-ganglioside antibodies as well as monoclonal antibodies raised against gangliosides induce neuronal cell lysis in culture by targeting specific cell surface gangliosides and this effect is complement dependent (Zhang *et al.*, 2004).

The GBS variant, acute motor axonal neuropathy (AMAN) has also been associated with anti-GM1, anti-GM1b, anti-GD1a, and anti-GalNAc-GD1a antibodies. The evidence for this is suggested by the finding that antibodies from patients have been shown to damage motor terminal endplates *in vitro* suggesting a pathogenic role in disease (Hughes and Cornblath, 2005).

Purified IgG from Miller-Fisher syndrome patients induced muscle weakness in adult mice due to inhibition of postsynaptic channels (Buchwald et al 1998). This effect was also seen with anti-GQ1b antibodies in conjunction with activated complement at the NMJ (Plomp *et al.*, 1999) while motor nerve terminal injury has also been shown to be associated with antibodies specific for disialoside epitopes on gangliosides GT1a (Halstead *et al.*, 2004).

ANIMAL MODELS OF GBS

As discussed above anti-GM1, anti-GM1b, anti-GD1a, and anti-GalNAc-GD1a IgG antibodies are associated with AMAN in humans. The antibodies have been shown to augment experimental autoimmune neuritis (EAN) in rabbits and induce clinical disease following immunization of rabbits with galactocerebrosides or GM1 ganglioside (Caporale *et al.*, 2006, Saida *et al.*, 1981). Paralyzed rabbits developed pathological changes in the peripheral nerves identical to changes seen in human GBS. Neurophysiological studies show that the anti-GM1 antibodies derived from immunised rabbits alter K- and Na-channels and disrupt the membrane at nodes of Ranvier (Takigawa *et al.*, 1995). The pathogenic role of antibodies to the ganglioside GD1b is evident from the induction of experimental sensory neuropathy in rabbits following immunization with GD1b (Kusunoki *et al.*, 1996; Kusunoki *et al.*, 1999). Animals developed experimental sensory ataxic neuropathy with severe axonal degeneration in the dorsal column, dorsal roots and sciatic nerve. Antibodies to GD1b bound to large primary sensory neurons and were considered the underlying cause of disease.

The axonal variant of GBS, AMAN, can also be modelled in rabbits following immunization with the lipo-oligosaccharide of *Campylobacter jejuni,* which, as mentioned above, induces antibodies cross-reacting with gangliosides (Yuki *et al.*, 2004). The immunogenicity these ganglioside epitopes in lipo-oligosaccharide of *C. jejuni* were also demonstrated following immunization of guinea pigs using the *C. jejuni* strain HB9313, which resulted in neuropathy and axonal degeneration (Shu *et al.*, 2006).

The development of mouse models for GBS and/or related disorders has proven to be more difficult as mice were shown to be tolerant for gangliosides (Bowes *et al.*, 2002). In this study it was shown that mice deficient for the enzyme GalNAc-transferase, which is necessary for the synthesis of complex gangliosides like GM1 and GD1a, produced higher levels of ganglioside-specific antibodies after immunisation than wild-type mice. The antibodies were pathogenic as determined using ex vivo diaphragm preparations that overexpress gangliosides which resulted in complement-mediated damage (Goodfellow *et al.*, 2005). In contrast, wild-type mice immunised with lipo-oligosaccharides derived from *C. jejuni* or from *Brucella melitensis* induce cross-reactive antibodies against gangliosides more easily (Bowes *et al.*, 2002, Watanabe *et al.*, 2005). The anti-GM1 ganglioside antibody response produced by BALB/c mice in response to *Brucella melitensis* was strong enough to result in flaccid limb weakness (Watanabe *et al.*, 2005). These studies suggest that lipo-oligosaccharides are more immunogenic than gangliosides; possibly this is related to the ability of lipo-oligosaccharides to activate the innate receptor toll-like receptor 4, which leads to release of pro-inflammatory cytokines (Kuijf *et al.*, 2010, Rathinam *et al.*, 2009).

In vivo monoclonal antibodies directed to gangliosides, transferred to mice as hybridomas induced axonal neuropathy affecting a small proportion of nerve fibres whereas purified anti-ganglioside antibodies had no effect despite high titre circulating antibodies (Sheikh *et al.*, 2004). It was suggested that this effect was due to properties of the hybridoma on the blood nerve barrier eg by allowing direct access of immunoglobulin to the nerve.

In conclusion, evidence for autoimmunity to neuronal antigens in GBS comes from the finding of autoantibodies in patients, passive transfer of antibodies to laboratory animals as well as experimental disease induced following active immunisation with neuronal antigens.

DIABETIC NEUROPATHY

In other autoimmune disorders such as diabetes antibodies to neuronal structures have also been described and are associated with peripheral neuropathies. Nearly 60% of all people with diabetes suffer from peripheral neuropathy in which the underlying mechanisms are unknown although autoimmune responses to neuronal structures may play a key role. Neurons and pancreatic Beta-cells share common determinants such as GAD. In early diabetes GAD specific antibodies are present and patients with high levels of GAD-65 antibodies were more likely to develop neuropathological complications. Although there is not a clear association between the presence of GAD65 antibodies and diabetic neuropathy autoantibodies were associated with worse peripheral nerve function (Hoeldtke *et al.*, 2000). Serum from diabetic type-1 patients react with neuroblastoma cells in culture and exert apoptotic effects on neurons in culture (Vinik *et al.*, 2005).

Using whole-cell recording of rat cerebellar slices it was shown that Ig in CSF from ataxic patients with anti-GAD antibodies reduced gamma-aminobutyric acid (GABA) in vitro (Mitoma *et al.*, 2003). More specifically the pathogenic role of anti-GAD Ig in the CSF in a patient with progressive cerebellar ataxia associated with insulin-dependent diabetes was clearly demonstrated by a selective suppression of the inhibitory postsynaptic currents in Purkinje cells (Ishida *et al.*, 2007). While the mechanism of neuronal damage is unclear, (Towns *et al.*, 2005) showed that serum from diabetic patients with neuropathy induced autophagy, a lysosome-dependent degradation pathway of cytoplasmic contents, in the neuronal SH-SY5Y cells. The effect was abolished when serum was incubated with Protein L beads, which bind immunoglobulin, suggesting that autophagy was induced by autoantibodies present in the patients' serum.

A neuronal autoantigen that has been identified in diabetic NOD mice is peripherin. This is a class III intermediate filament that is expressed predominantly in axons of the peripheral nervous system but also in pancreatic Beta cells. Peripherin reactivity was found in pancreatic islet-infiltrating B cells of the mice (Puertas *et al.*, 2007). Recently peripherin-reactive antibodies were also detected in humans and were associated with autonomic dysfunction or endocrinopathy, including diabetes (Chamberlain *et al.*, 2010).

ANIMAL MODELS OF DIABETIC NEUROPATHY

Mechanisms underlying the neurological complications in diabetic patients have been studied in the experimental models of diabetes namely non-obese diabetic (NOD), streptozotocin (STZ)-induced diabetic mice (type 1 diabetes), db/db mouse (type 2 diabetes) and diabetic BBW rats (Calcutt, 2002, Schmidt *et al.*, 2003). As well as diabetes these animals also develop neuropathy similar to diabetic patients providing a model to study mechanism of disease. While the role of antibodies in neuropathy is unknown autoreactive T cells are observed in the peripheral nerves although neuropathy is not dependent perforin or fas pathways (Bour-Jordan *et al.*, 2005).

MONOCLONAL GAMMOPATHY

Antibodies to neurofilament proteins have been associated with a variety of disorders including neuropathy with monoclonal gammopathy of undetermined significance (MGUS). In these patients antibodies to NF-heavy in the serum bind to neuronal antigens (Stubbs *et al.*, 2003). The pathogenic potential of serum containing NF antibodies was demonstrated following injection of rat sciatic nerve. Serum containing antibodies to NF but not control serum altered the axonal calibre and induced vesiculation and ovoid formation leading to peripheral nerve conduction block (Stubbs *et al.*, 2003). Furthermore patients with slowly progressive sensory motor axonal neuropathology were shown to have a monoclonal IgG-kappa that bound to NF protein (Nemni *et al.*, 1990), however the pathogenic significance of this M-protein was not established.

Thus in some peripheral neuropathies it is clear that infectious agents are associated with the neurological disease due to induction of autoimmune responses to neuronal antigens. These studies highlight the strong link between such autoimmune responses and neuronal damage.

REFERENCES

Bae JS and Kim BJ 2005. Cerebellar ataxia and acute motor axonal neuropathy associated with Anti GD1b and Anti GM1 antibodies. *J. Clin. Neurosci.* 12: 808-10.

Bour-Jordan H, Thompson HL and Bluestone JA 2005. Distinct effector mechanisms in the development of autoimmune neuropathy versus diabetes in nonobese diabetic mice. *J. Immunol.* 175: 5649-55.

Bowes T, Wagner ER, Boffey J, Nicholl D, Cochrane L, Benboubetra M, Conner J, Furukawa K and Willison HJ 2002. Tolerance to self gangliosides is the major factor restricting the antibody response to lipopolysaccharide core oligosaccharides in Campylobacter jejuni strains associated with Guillain-Barre syndrome. *Infect. Immun.* 70: 5008-18.

Calcutt NA 2002. Future treatments for diabetic neuropathy: clues from experimental neuropathy. *Curr. Diab. Rep.* 2: 482-8.

Caporale CM, Capasso M, Luciani M, Prencipe V, Creati B, Gandolfi P, De Angelis MV, Di Muzio A, Caporale V and Uncini A 2006. Experimental axonopathy induced by immunization with Campylobacter jejuni lipopolysaccharide from a patient with Guillain-Barre syndrome. *J. Neuroimmunol.* 174: 12-20.

Chamberlain JL, Pittock SJ, Oprescu AM, Dege C, Apiwattanakul M, Kryzer TJ and Lennon VA 2010. Peripherin-IgG association with neurologic and endocrine autoimmunity. *J. Autoimmun.* 34: 469-77.

Gong Y, Tagawa Y, Lunn MP, Laroy W, Heffer-Lauc M, Li CY, Griffin JW, Schnaar RL and Sheikh KA 2002. Localization of major gangliosides in the PNS: implications for immune neuropathies. *Brain.* 125: 2491-506.

Goodfellow JA, Bowes T, Sheikh K, Odaka M, Halstead SK, Humphreys PD, Wagner ER, Yuki N, Furukawa K, Plomp JJ and Willison HJ 2005. Overexpression of GD1a ganglioside sensitizes motor nerve terminals to anti-GD1a antibody-mediated injury in a model of acute motor axonal neuropathy. *J. Neurosci.* 25: 1620-8.

Greenshields KN, Halstead SK, Zitman FM, Rinaldi S, Brennan KM, O'Leary C, Chamberlain LH, Easton A, Roxburgh J, Pediani J, Furukawa K, Goodyear CS, Plomp JJ and Willison HJ 2009. The neuropathic potential of anti-GM1 autoantibodies is regulated by the local glycolipid environment in mice. *J. Clin. Invest.* 119: 595-610.

Halstead SK, O'Hanlon GM, Humphreys PD, Morrison DB, Morgan BP, Todd AJ, Plomp JJ and Willison HJ 2004. Anti-disialoside antibodies kill perisynaptic Schwann cells and damage motor nerve terminals via membrane attack complex in a murine model of neuropathy. *Brain.* 127: 2109-23.

Hoeldtke RD, Bryner KD, Hobbs GR, Horvath GG, Riggs JE, Christie I, Ganser G, Marcovina SM and Lernmark A 2000. Antibodies to glutamic acid decarboxylase and peripheral nerve function in type 1 diabetes. *J. Clin. Endocrinol. Metab.* 85: 3297-308.

Hughes RA and Cornblath DR 2005. Guillain-Barre syndrome. *Lancet.* 366: 1653-66.

Ishida K, Mitoma H, Wada Y, Oka T, Shibahara J, Saito Y, Murayama S and Mizusawa H 2007. Selective loss of Purkinje cells in a patient with anti-glutamic acid decarboxylase antibody-associated cerebellar ataxia. *J. Neurol. Neurosurg. Psychiatry.* 78: 190-2.

Jacobs BC, Rothbarth PH, van der Meche FG, Herbrink P, Schmitz PI, de Klerk MA and van Doorn PA 1998. The spectrum of antecedent infections in Guillain-Barre syndrome: a case-control study. *Neurology.* 51: 1110-5.

Kaida K, Morita D, Kanzaki M, Kamakura K, Motoyoshi K, Hirakawa M and Kusunoki S 2004. Ganglioside complexes as new target antigens in Guillain-Barre syndrome. *Ann. Neurol.* 56: 567-71.

Koga M, Yoshino H, Morimatsu M and Yuki N 2002. Anti-GT1a IgG in Guillain-Barre syndrome. *J. Neurol. Neurosurg. Psychiatry.* 72: 767-71.

Kuijf ML, Samsom JN, van Rijs W, Bax M, Huizinga R, Heikema AP, van Doorn PA, van Belkum A, van Kooyk Y, Burgers PC, Luider TM, Endtz HP, Nieuwenhuis EE and Jacobs BC 2010. TLR4-mediated sensing of Campylobacter jejuni by dendritic cells is determined by sialylation. *J. Immunol.* 185: 748-55.

Kusunoki S, Hitoshi S, Kaida K, Arita M and Kanazawa I 1999. Monospecific anti-GD1b IgG is required to induce rabbit ataxic neuropathy. *Ann. Neurol.* 45: 400-3.

Kusunoki S, Shimizu J, Chiba A, Ugawa Y, Hitoshi S and Kanazawa I 1996. Experimental sensory neuropathy induced by sensitization with ganglioside GD1b. *Ann. Neurol.* 39: 424-31.

Liu JX, Willison HJ and Pedrosa-Domellof F 2009. Immunolocalization of GQ1b and related gangliosides in human extraocular neuromuscular junctions and muscle spindles. *Invest. Ophthalmol. Vis Sci* 50: 3226-32.

Mitoma H, Ishida K, Shizuka-Ikeda M and Mizusawa H 2003. Dual impairment of GABAA- and GABAB-receptor-mediated synaptic responses by autoantibodies to glutamic acid decarboxylase. *J. Neurol. Sci.* 208: 51-6.

Nemni R, Feltri ML, Fazio R, Quattrini A, Lorenzetti I, Corbo M and Canal N 1990. Axonal neuropathy with monoclonal IgG kappa that binds to a neurofilament protein. *Ann. Neurol.* 28: 361-4.

Plomp JJ, Molenaar PC, O'Hanlon GM, Jacobs BC, Veitch J, Daha MR, van Doorn PA, van der Meche FG, Vincent A, Morgan BP and Willison HJ

1999. Miller Fisher anti-GQ1b antibodies: alpha-latrotoxin-like effects on motor end plates. *Ann. Neurol.* 45: 189-99.

Puertas MC, Carrillo J, Pastor X, Ampudia RM, Planas R, Alba A, Bruno R, Pujol-Borrell R, Estanyol JM, Vives-Pi M and Verdaguer J 2007. Peripherin is a relevant neuroendocrine autoantigen recognized by islet-infiltrating B lymphocytes. *J. Immunol.* 178: 6533-9.

Rathinam VA, Appledorn DM, Hoag KA, Amalfitano A and Mansfield LS 2009. Campylobacter jejuni-induced activation of dendritic cells involves cooperative signaling through Toll-like receptor 4 (TLR4)-MyD88 and TLR4-TRIF axes. *Infect. Immun.* 77: 2499-507.

Saida T, Saida K, Silberberg DH and Brown MJ 1981. Experimental allergic neuritis induced by galactocerebroside. *Ann. Neurol.* 9 Suppl: 87-101.

Schmidt RE, Dorsey DA, Beaudet LN and Peterson RG 2003. Analysis of the Zucker Diabetic Fatty (ZDF) type 2 diabetic rat model suggests a neurotrophic role for insulin/IGF-I in diabetic autonomic neuropathy. *Am. J. Pathol.* 163: 21-8.

Sheikh KA, Zhang G, Gong Y, Schnaar RL and Griffin JW 2004. An anti-ganglioside antibody-secreting hybridoma induces neuropathy in mice. *Ann. Neurol.* 56: 228-39.

Shu XM, Cai FC and Zhang XP 2006. Carbohydrate mimicry of Campylobacter jejuni lipooligosaccharide is critical for the induction of anti-GM1 antibody and neuropathy. *Muscle Nerve.* 33: 225-31.

Stubbs EB, Jr., Lawlor MW, Richards MP, Siddiqui K, Fisher MA, Bhoopalam N and Siegel GJ 2003. Anti-neurofilament antibodies in neuropathy with monoclonal gammopathy of undetermined significance produce experimental motor nerve conduction block. *Acta Neuropathol. (Berl)* 105: 109-16.

Susuki K, Yuki N and Hirata K 2001. Features of sensory ataxic neuropathy associated with anti-GD1b IgM antibody. *J. Neuroimmunol.* 112: 181-7.

Takigawa T, Yasuda H, Kikkawa R, Shigeta Y, Saida T and Kitasato H 1995. Antibodies against GM1 ganglioside affect K+ and Na+ currents in isolated rat myelinated nerve fibers. *Ann. Neurol.* 37: 436-42.

Towns R, Kabeya Y, Yoshimori T, Guo C, Shangguan Y, Hong S, Kaplan M, Klionsky DJ and Wiley JW 2005. Sera from patients with type 2 diabetes and neuropathy induce autophagy and colocalization with mitochondria in SY5Y cells. *Autophagy.* 1: 163-70.

Vinik AI, Anandacoomaraswamy D and Ullal J 2005. Antibodies to neuronal structures: innocent bystanders or neurotoxins? *Diabetes Care.* 28: 2067-72.

Watanabe K, Kim S, Nishiguchi M, Suzuki H and Watarai M 2005. Brucella melitensis infection associated with Guillain-Barre syndrome through molecular mimicry of host structures. *FEMS Immunol. Med. Microbiol.* 45: 121-7.

Yuki N, Susuki K, Koga M, Nishimoto Y, Odaka M, Hirata K, Taguchi K, Miyatake T, Furukawa K, Kobata T and Yamada M 2004. Carbohydrate mimicry between human ganglioside GM1 and Campylobacter jejuni lipooligosaccharide causes Guillain-Barre syndrome. *Proc. Natl. Acad. Sci. U. S. A.* 101: 11404-9.

Zhang G, Lopez PH, Li CY, Mehta NR, Griffin JW, Schnaar RL and Sheikh KA 2004. Anti-ganglioside antibody-mediated neuronal cytotoxicity and its protection by intravenous immunoglobulin: implications for immune neuropathies. *Brain.* 127: 1085-100.

Chapter 4

PARANEOPLASTIC NEUROLOGICAL DISORDERS

Ruth Huizinga[1] and Sandra Amor[2,3]

[1] Department of Immunology, Erasmus MC,
University Medical Center, Rotterdam, The Netherlands.
[2] Department of Pathology, VU Medical Center Amsterdam,
The Netherlands.
[3] Neuroscience and Trauma Centre,
Barts and the London School of Medicine and Dentistry,
Queen Mary University of London, United Kingdom.

INTRODUCTION

The paraneoplastic neurological disorders (PND) are observed in patients who have cancer along with abnormal neurological symptoms despite the absence of tumours in the nervous system. Common tumours of the breast, ovary and lung express several proteins generally restricted to the nervous system and, as a consequence patients generate immune responses to these 'nervous system specific' proteins. While autoimmune responses to these neuronal antigens help to suppress the growth of the tumour they also cause damage in the nervous system leading to neurological symptoms (Dalmau and Rosenfeld, 2008, Didelot and Honnorat, 2009). PND are thus considered to be due to autoimmune attack on neurons expressing the antigens abnormally expressed by the tumour. The clinical syndromes are very heterogeneous due to the many different regions of the nervous system that may be involved (Table 2) although it should be noted that for many PND the neuronal antigen expressed by the tumour is unknown. In many of these disorders antibodies against the tumour and the neurons are detected in the patient's serum and cerebrospinal fluid (Posner, 2003).

The majority of the PND antigens are intracellular and are thus not readily available for recognition by antibodies although, as demonstrated in other pathological conditions, antibodies do gain access to intracellular proteins. Indeed PND antibodies enter neurons and may trigger responses in the neuron such as apoptosis. Alternatively, CD8+ cytotoxic T cells may be activated by dendritic cells that have taken up tumour cells in the periphery and cross present not only tumour antigens but also the neuronal antigens. In this way the CD8+ cytotoxic T cells not only respond to the tumour but could recognise and thus target neurons (Albert *et al.*, 1998). In the following sections we will briefly summarise the most common PND, after which we will discuss the pathogenic role of anti-neuronal antibodies and T cells as evidenced by studies in patients and animals.

SUBACUTE SENSORY NEUROPATHY

Subacute sensory neuropathy (SSN), or anti-Hu syndrome, is associated with anti-Hu antibodies that recognize anti-neuronal nuclear antigen-1 (ANNA-1), an RNA binding proteins. This disease typically involves dorsal root ganglia, where cell bodies of sensory neurons degenerate. Symptoms include numbness, sensory ataxia, pain and weakness, often with an asymmetric onset (Rudnicki and Dalmau, 2005). Other regions of the CNS and PNS may also be affected, explaining the occurrence of motor symptoms (Camdessanche *et al.*, 2002). SSN is typically associated with small cell lung carcinoma and anti-Hu antibodies. The association of SSN with breast, ovarian and prostate tumours partly explains the finding of other paraneoplastic antibodies including anti-CRMP-5 (cytoplasmic collapsin response mediated protein-5) and anti-amphiphysin (Pittock *et al.*, 2005, Yu *et al.*, 2001). On the other hand, the percentage of patients with anti-Hu antibodies who do not have concomitant cancer is less than 2% (Graus *et al.*, 2004).

PARANEOPLASTIC CEREBELLAR DEGENERATION

In paraneoplastic cerebellar degeneration (PCD), autoimmune responses to antigens of cerebellar Purkinje neurons are expressed by breast or ovarian tumour. The so-called anti-Yo antibodies typically found in these patients are directed against cerebellar degeneration-related protein-2 (cdr-2), a cytoplasmic protein expressed in cerebellar Purkinje cells. Antibodies to voltage-gated calcium channels (VGCC) have also been demonstrated in patients with cerebellar degeneration associated with lung cancer (Graus *et al.*, 2002). Pathogenic effects of VGCC-reactive antibodies have been demonstrated in the context of Lambert-Eaton myasthenic syndrome (LEMS; see chapter 2). Finally, PCD can be induced by Hodgkin's disease and is associated with antibodies to Tr, which is expressed in the cytoplasm of Purkinje cells, and with antibodies to the metabotropic glutamate receptor type I (mGluR1) (Bernal *et al.*, 2003, Sillevis Smitt *et al.*, 2000).

LIMBIC ENCEPHALITIS

Limbic encephalitis is a rare disorder of the CNS in which patients suffer from memory deficits, seizures and personality changes. Diagnosis is often difficult as the symptoms are frequently observed in association with other conditions and because the neurological symptoms can precede the detection of cancer. Limbic encephalitis predominantly occurs in conjunction with small cell carcinomas of the lung and testicular tumours, which induce production of anti-Hu and anti-Ma2 antibodies (also referred to as anti-Ta) (Gultekin *et al.*, 2000). As in patients with neuromyotonia, antibodies to VGKC-associated proteins have been detected in limbic encephalitis. Those antigens include contactin-associated protein-2 (caspr) and leucin-rich glioma inactivated 1 protein (Irani *et al.*, 2010). In contrast to other paraneoplastic disorders of the CNS, limbic encephalitis associated with antibodies to VGKC is is more often sensitive to immunotherapy (Thieben *et al.*, 2004).

Table 1. Paraneoplastic neurological disorders – associations with antineuronal antibodies

Antigens	Antibody	Expression, distribution and role	Neurological disease association	Tumor	Reference
Hu antigens [HuB, HuC, HuD (Hel-N1)	Anti-Hu (ANNA-1)	35–40 kDa neuron specific RNA binding proteins	SSN Limbic encephalitis	SCLC	Tanaka 2004 Rousseau et al., 2005
Yo (PCA-1; cdr-2)	Anti-Yo	Purkinje cells; 62 kDa intracellular protein; binds to myc	PCD	Ovarian & breast carcinomas	Tanaka 2004
Ri (genes Nova-1 and Nova-2)	anti-Ri (ANNA-2)	Neuronal nuclei; 55 and 80kDa neuron specific RNA binding proteins	Opsoclonus myoclonus ataxia	SCLC, breast carcinoma	Fadare and Hart 2004
Ma antigens [Ma1 (PNMA1), Ma2 (Ta, PNMA2), Ma3 (PNMA3)	Anti-Ma1 Anti-Ma2 / Ta Anti-Ma3	Ma-1 37kDa neuron and testis Ma-2 40 kDa neurons of limbic system	Limbic encephalitis	SCLC, testis	Gultekin et al., 2000
CRMP-5	Anti-CRMP-5	62 kd neuronal cytoplasmic protein	PCD	SCLC thymoma	Yu et al., 2001
ANNA-3	ANNA-3	170 kDa in nuclei of Purkinje cells	PCD Limbic encephalitis	SCLC	(Chan et al., 2001)
Tr	Anti-Tr	Purkinje cells; cytosol and outer surface of ER	Tr syndrome	Hodgkin's lymphoma	Bernal et al., 2003

Antigens	Antibody	Expression, distribution and role	Neurological disease association	Tumor	Reference
Amphiphysin	Anti-amphiphysin	128kDa pre-synaptic nerve terminal protein	Stiff person syndrome	Lung and thymoma	Folli *et al.*, 1993
AChR	Anti-AChR	Transmembrane protein; neuromuscular junction	Myasthenia gravis	Thymoma	(Vincent, 2006)
VGCC	Anti-VGCC	Presynaptic ion channel; neuromuscular junction and cerebellum	PCD LEMS	SCLC	Graus *et al.*, 2002 Vincent, 2006
mGluR1	Anti-mGluR1	Cerebellar Purkinje cells, cerebellar cortex	PCD	Hodgkin's lymphoma	Coesmans *et al.*, 2003

Abbreviations: AChR, acetyl choline receptor; LEMS, Lambert-Eaton myasthenic syndrome; PCD, paraneoplastic cerebellar degeneration; SCLC, small cell lung carcinoma; SSN, subacute sensory neuronopathy; VGCC, voltage gated calcium channels; VGKC, voltage gated potassium channels.

OPSOCLONUS MYOCLONUS

Opsoclonus myoclonus is a paraneoplastic disorder characterised by rapid involuntary eye movements as well as muscle contractions (hence also referred to as dancing eye syndrome). In approximately 50% of children with the disease an underlying neuroblastoma can be detected. In adults, opsoclonus myoclonus is associated with lung and ovarian cancers and in some cases with autoantibodies to Ri. The antigen Ri encoded by the gene *Nova* is expressed in the brain stem, cortex and motor neurons, and also by lung and ovarian tumors (Fadare and Hart, 2004). Children with opsoclonus muoclonus have IgG antibodies that bind surface membrane antigens on neuroblastoma cells and induce apoptosis, however the exact antigens remain to be identified (Blaes *et al.*, 2005, Korfei *et al.*, 2005). In addition to a paraneoplastic aetiology, opsoclonus myoclonus may follow a viral infection but has, similar to basal ganglia disease, also been reported following pharyngitis due to streptococcal infection in which the antigen was identified as neuroleukin (Candler *et al.*, 2006).

STIFF PERSON SYNDROME

The Stiff Person Syndrome (SPS) is a chronic neurological disorder characterized by progressive stiffness, painful persistent or spasmodic muscle contractions, mostly involving spine and lower extremities. Paraneoplastic forms of SPS are characterised by the presence of antibodies to amphiphysin, a protein involved in clathrin-mediated endocytosis (Folli *et al.*, 1993). Non-paraneoplastic forms of SPS are associated with the presence of autoantibodies against glutamic acid decarboxylase (GAD), an enzyme that converts the excitatory neurotransmitter glutamate to gamma-aminobutyric acid (GABA), a major inhibitory neurotransmitter of the CNS. The syndrome often occurs spontaneously and in association with type I (insulin-dependent) diabetes mellitus (Schloot *et al.*, 1999). The relevant treatment for SPS is to alter the inhibitory processes controlling muscle activity, control of the immune response and removal of associated neoplasia. High-dose intravenous immunoglobulin (IVIg) has been shown to be effective suggesting an involvement of humoral immunity in disease.

OTHER PARANEOPLASTIC DISORDERS

Paraneoplastic syndromes also affect the lower motor neurons as described in a patient with breast cancer with antibodies directed against axons and nodes of Ranvier. More detailed studies showed that these antibodies were directed to isoforms of βIV spectrin – a protein enriched in axonal initial segments and nodes of Ranvier (Berghs *et al.*, 2001). Finally, myasthenia gravis is in some cases associated with thymoma (see chapter 2).

ROLE OF ANTIBODIES IN PND

Compared to autoimmune diseases of the neuromuscular junction, like myasthenia gravis, most neoplastic antigens in PND are intracellular antigens and were thus considered unlikely to be targeted by the antibody directly. It is probably for this reason that development of models or demonstration for a direct pathogenic effect of antibodies has been difficult. Nevertheless some PND can be treated with IVIg suggesting that antibodies do play a role at least in some forms of PND (Vincent *et al.*, 2010).

Many studies reported that anti-Yo antibodies were not pathogenic. For example, application of anti-Yo or anti-Hu antibodies on primary mouse-brain-derived neurons did not kill neurons, but instead induced the expression of cell adhesion molecules and accelerated neuronal differentiation. Similar effects of serum IgG fractions from patients containing the anti-Yo or the anti-Hu antibody on the cultured neurons were observed, suggesting that their effects were not through the binding of the antibody to specific antigens, but to some other factors contained in IgG fractions (Tanaka *et al.*, 2004). Recently, rat organotypic slice cultures have been used to determine the pathogenicity of anti-Yo antibodies. Administration of the antibodies resulted in uptake and accumulation in Purkinje cells and was associated with neuronal cell death (Greenlee *et al.*, 2010). Control IgG was also taken up by Purkinje cells but did not accumulate (Hill *et al.*, 2009). Likewise, IgG purified from the serum of patients with Hodgkin's disease in relation to PCD in which the number of Purkinje cells is severely reduced was shown to affect the basal activity of Purkinje cells in mouse brain slice cultures (Coesmans *et al.*, 2003).

The role of anti-GAD antibodies in SPS is still unclear although decreased GABA synthesis in nerve terminals as a result of antibody interference with exocytosis of GABA may be crucial to disease expression. This is suggested from *in vitro* studies whereby GAD autoantibodies or purified IgG from the

CSF or serum from people with SPS were observed to reduce GABA production in crude rat cerebellar extracts (Dinkel *et al.*, 1998).

ROLE OF T CELLS IN PND

Autoreactive cytotoxic T lymphocytes (CTLs) specific for a cytoplasmic protein of Purkinje cells cdr2 are present in the blood of patients with PCD (Albert *et al.*, 1998), suggesting that they may play a role in the ensuing neuronal damage. CD8+ T cells were detected in the dentate gyrus, but not in the cerebellum of a patient with PCD (Aye *et al.*, 2009). Likewise T cell responses to Hu-D peptides are present in patients with neuronal and axonal injury particularly those with the anti-Hu syndrome (Rousseau *et al.*, 2005), although others have not been able to detect such responses (de Beukelaar *et al.*, 2007). Analysis of the T cell receptor repertoire of T cells in CNS tissues of patients with sensory neuronopathy is in favour of an oligoclonal T cell response to onconeural antigens (Voltz *et al.*, 1998). The pathological significance of such responses was demonstrated by lysis of autologous fibroblasts by activated CD8+ T cells from a patient following induced expression of HLA class I and HuD protein on the fibroblasts (Tanaka *et al.*, 1999). These authors also demonstrated cytotoxic T cell activity to Yo protein expressed by autologous dendritic cells suggesting that cytotoxic T cells could be involved in Purkinje cell loss in paraneoplastic cerebellar degeneration (Tanaka *et al.*, 1998).

ANIMAL MODELS FOR PND

The number of studies demonstrating the pathogenic effects of antibodies to intracellular paraneoplastic neuroantigens is scarce however early studies show that microinjection of anti-Yo antibodies from humans in rats reach the CNS (Greenlee *et al.*, 1995). While anti-Yo antibodies were identified on the dendrites and within the cell body of Purkinje cells, animals did not develop ataxia or cerebellar injury. Additional studies to determine the mechanism of action are required to provide clues to their effect in human disease. As mentioned before, the anti-Yo antibodies recognise the antigen cdr2 on Purkinje cells. By immunising mice with naked cdr2 cDNA autoantibodies against Purkinje cells could be induced and CTLs from these mice lysed cells pulsed with H-2K-restricted cdr2 peptide, however clinical or pathological changes in the cerebellum were absent (Sakai et al., 2001). Earlier studies also showed that immunization with recombinant Yo protein did not cause damage to Purkinje cells (Tanaka et al., 1995).

Immunization of mice with a plasmid coding HuD induced a strong and specific anti-Hu response. To model the human disease mice were challenged by implantation of a neuroblastoma cell line that constitutively expresses HuD. In the presence of secreted HuD and subsequent immunity to Hu significant inhibition of tumour growth was observed however the animals did not develop neurological deficits or neuropathological evidence of nervous system pathology (Carpentier et al., 1998, Sillevis Smitt et al., 1996). Possibly, this may be related to the fact that HuD-specific T cells of normal mice can not be activated in vivo, in contrast to HuD null mice, in which HuD-specific T cells can be expanded (DeLuca et al., 2009). This study indicates that T cells under normal circumstances are tolerant to the HuD antigen.

Development of animal models for PND has focussed on induction of antibodies to onconeuroantigens and as such has been problematic. As a step to study the involvement of T cells in PND, (Pellkofer et al., 2004) show that following immunisation of rats with Ma1, transfer of T-cell blasts specific from the rats into naïve animals induced encephalitis indicating a role for T cells in PND. However, animals did not develop clinical disease.

The most compelling evidence for a pathogenic role for paraneoplastic antibodies is based on studies with IgG antibodies to the intracellular synaptic protein amphiphysin purified from patients with SPS. The antibodies recognised rat CNS tissue and when injected intraperitoneally, induced stiffness with spasms in rats (Sommer et al., 2005). It is important to mention that in this particular study, MBP reactive T cells were co-transferred to open the blood brain barrier and that high and repeated doses of antibodies were required to induce the clinical signs. In a follow-up study anti-amphiphysin antibodies were injected intrathecally into rats and were found to be internalised by neurons, an effect that was not observed in amphiphysin knockout mice. The antibodies subsequently interfered with vesicular endocytosis, especially in GABAergic synapses, resulting in decreased inhibitory currents (Geis et al., 2010). Together these studies elegantly show that in SPS patients, antibodies to neuronal antigens not only induced physiological changes in vitro but also mimic the human disease in experimental animals. It remains to be seen whether immunization of experimental animals with amphiphysin leads to clinical disease as observed in patients.

REFERENCES

Albert ML, Darnell JC, Bender A, Francisco LM, Bhardwaj N and Darnell RB 1998. Tumor-specific killer cells in paraneoplastic cerebellar degeneration. *Nat. Med.* 4: 1321-4.

Aye MM, Kasai T, Tashiro Y, Xing HQ, Shirahama H, Mitsuda M, Suetsugu T, Tanaka K, Osame M and Izumo S 2009. CD8 positive T-cell infiltration in the dentate nucleus of paraneoplastic cerebellar degeneration. *J. Neuroimmunol.* 208: 136-40.

Berghs S, Ferracci F, Maksimova E, Gleason S, Leszczynski N, Butler M, De Camilli P and Solimena M 2001. Autoimmunity to beta IV spectrin in paraneoplastic lower motor neuron syndrome. *Proc. Natl. Acad. Sci. U. S. A.* 98: 6945-50.

Bernal F, Shams'ili S, Rojas I, Sanchez-Valle R, Saiz A, Dalmau J, Honnorat J, Sillevis Smitt P and Graus F 2003. Anti-Tr antibodies as markers of paraneoplastic cerebellar degeneration and Hodgkin's disease. *Neurology.* 60: 230-4.

Blaes F, Fuhlhuber V, Korfei M, Tschernatsch M, Behnisch W, Rostasy K, Hero B, Kaps M and Preissner KT 2005. Surface-binding autoantibodies to cerebellar neurons in opsoclonus syndrome. Ann. Neurol. 58: 313-7.

Camdessanche JP, Antoine JC, Honnorat J, Vial C, Petiot P, Convers P and Michel D 2002. Paraneoplastic peripheral neuropathy associated with anti-Hu antibodies. A clinical and electrophysiological study of 20 patients. *Brain.* 125: 166-75.

Candler PM, Dale RC, Griffin S, Church AJ, Wait R, Chapman MD, Keir G, Giovannoni G and Rees JH 2006. Post-streptococcal opsoclonus-myoclonus syndrome associated with anti-neuroleukin antibodies. *J. Neurol. Neurosurg. Psychiatry.* 77: 507-12.

Carpentier AF, Rosenfeld MR, Delattre JY, Whalen RG, Posner JB and Dalmau J 1998. DNA vaccination with HuD inhibits growth of a neuroblastoma in mice. *Clin. Cancer Res.* 4: 2819-24.

Chan KH, Vernino S and Lennon VA 2001. ANNA-3 anti-neuronal nuclear antibody: marker of lung cancer-related autoimmunity. *Ann. Neurol.* 50: 301-11.

Coesmans M, Smitt PA, Linden DJ, Shigemoto R, Hirano T, Yamakawa Y, van Alphen AM, Luo C, van der Geest JN, Kros JM, Gaillard CA, Frens MA and de Zeeuw CI 2003. Mechanisms underlying cerebellar motor deficits due to mGluR1-autoantibodies. *Ann. Neurol.* 53: 325-36.

Dalmau J and Rosenfeld MR 2008. Paraneoplastic syndromes of the CNS. *Lancet Neurol.* 7: 327-40.

de Beukelaar JW, Verjans GM, van Norden Y, Milikan JC, Kraan J, Hooijkaas H, Sintnicolaas K, Gratama JW and Sillevis Smitt PA 2007. No evidence for circulating HuD-specific CD8+ T cells in patients with paraneoplastic neurological syndromes and Hu antibodies. *Cancer Immunol. Immunother.* 56: 1501-6.

DeLuca I, Blachere NE, Santomasso B and Darnell RB 2009. Tolerance to the neuron-specific paraneoplastic HuD antigen. *PLoS One.* 4: e5739.

Didelot A and Honnorat J 2009. Update on paraneoplastic neurological syndromes. *Curr. Opin. Oncol.* 21: 566-72.

Dinkel K, Meinck HM, Jury KM, Karges W and Richter W 1998. Inhibition of gamma-aminobutyric acid synthesis by glutamic acid decarboxylase autoantibodies in stiff-man syndrome. *Ann. Neurol.* 44: 194-201.

Fadare O and Hart HJ 2004. Anti-Ri antibodies associated with short-term memory deficits and a mature cystic teratoma of the ovary. *Int. Semin. Surg. Oncol.* 1: 11.

Folli F, Solimena M, Cofiell R, Austoni M, Tallini G, Fassetta G, Bates D, Cartlidge N, Bottazzo GF, Piccolo G and et al. 1993. Autoantibodies to a 128-kd synaptic protein in three women with the stiff-man syndrome and breast cancer. *N. Engl. J. Med.* 328: 546-51.

Geis C, Weishaupt A, Hallermann S, Grunewald B, Wessig C, Wultsch T, Reif A, Byts N, Beck M, Jablonka S, Boettger MK, Uceyler N, Fouquet W, Gerlach M, Meinck HM, Siren AL, Sigrist SJ, Toyka KV, Heckmann M and Sommer C 2010. Stiff person syndrome-associated autoantibodies to amphiphysin mediate reduced GABAergic inhibition. *Brain.*133: 3166-80.

Graus F, Delattre JY, Antoine JC, Dalmau J, Giometto B, Grisold W, Honnorat J, Smitt PS, Vedeler C, Verschuuren JJ, Vincent A and Voltz R 2004. Recommended diagnostic criteria for paraneoplastic neurological syndromes. *J. Neurol. Neurosurg. Psychiatry.* 75: 1135-40.

Graus F, Lang B, Pozo-Rosich P, Saiz A, Casamitjana R and Vincent A 2002. P/Q type calcium-channel antibodies in paraneoplastic cerebellar degeneration with lung cancer. *Neurology.* 59: 764-6.

Greenlee JE, Burns JB, Rose JW, Jaeckle KA and Clawson S 1995. Uptake of systemically administered human anticerebellar antibody by rat Purkinje cells following blood-brain barrier disruption. *Acta Neuropathol.* 89: 341-5.

Greenlee JE, Clawson SA, Hill KE, Wood BL, Tsunoda I and Carlson NG 2010. Purkinje cell death after uptake of anti-Yo antibodies in cerebellar slice cultures. *J. Neuropathol. Exp. Neurol.* 69: 997-1007.

Gultekin SH, Rosenfeld MR, Voltz R, Eichen J, Posner JB and Dalmau J 2000. Paraneoplastic limbic encephalitis: neurological symptoms, immunological findings and tumour association in 50 patients. *Brain.* 123 (Pt 7): 1481-94.

Hill KE, Clawson SA, Rose JW, Carlson NG and Greenlee JE 2009. Cerebellar Purkinje cells incorporate immunoglobulins and immunotoxins in vitro: implications for human neurological disease and immunotherapeutics. *J. Neuroinflammation.* 6: 31.

Irani SR, Alexander S, Waters P, Kleopa KA, Pettingill P, Zuliani L, Peles E, Buckley C, Lang B and Vincent A 2010. Antibodies to Kv1 potassium channel-complex proteins leucine-rich, glioma inactivated 1 protein and contactin-associated protein-2 in limbic encephalitis, Morvan's syndrome and acquired neuromyotonia. *Brain.* 133: 2734-48.

Korfei M, Fuhlhuber V, Schmidt-Woll T, Kaps M, Preissner KT and Blaes F 2005. Functional characterisation of autoantibodies from patients with pediatric opsoclonus-myoclonus-syndrome. *J. Neuroimmunol.* 170: 150-7.

Pellkofer H, Schubart AS, Hoftberger R, Schutze N, Pagany M, Schuller M, Lassmann H, Hohlfeld R, Voltz R and Linington C 2004. Modelling paraneoplastic CNS disease: T-cells specific for the onconeuronal antigen PNMA1 mediate autoimmune encephalomyelitis in the rat. *Brain.* 127: 1822-30.

Pittock SJ, Lucchinetti CF, Parisi JE, Benarroch EE, Mokri B, Stephan CL, Kim KK, Kilimann MW and Lennon VA 2005. Amphiphysin autoimmunity: paraneoplastic accompaniments. *Ann. Neurol.* 58: 96-107.

Posner JB 2003. Immunology of paraneoplastic syndromes: overview. *Ann. N. Y. Acad. Sci.* 998: 178-86.

Rousseau A, Benyahia B, Dalmau J, Connan F, Guillet JG, Delattre JY and Choppin J 2005. T cell response to Hu-D peptides in patients with anti-Hu syndrome. *J. Neurooncol.* 71: 231-6.

Rudnicki SA and Dalmau J 2005. Paraneoplastic syndromes of the peripheral nerves. *Curr. Opin. Neurol.* 18: 598-603.

Sakai K, Shirakawa T, Kitagawa Y, Li Y and Hirose G 2001. Induction of cytotoxic T lymphocytes specific for paraneoplastic cerebellar degeneration-associated antigen in vivo by DNA immunization. *J. Autoimmun.* 17: 297-302.

Schloot NC, Batstra MC, Duinkerken G, De Vries RR, Dyrberg T, Chaudhuri A, Behan PO and Roep BO 1999. GAD65-Reactive T cells in a non-diabetic stiff-man syndrome patient. *J. Autoimmun.* 12: 289-96.

Sillevis Smitt P, Kinoshita A, De Leeuw B, Moll W, Coesmans M, Jaarsma D, Henzen-Logmans S, Vecht C, De Zeeuw C, Sekiyama N, Nakanishi S and Shigemoto R 2000. Paraneoplastic cerebellar ataxia due to autoantibodies against a glutamate receptor. *N. Engl. J. Med.* 342: 21-7.

Sillevis Smitt P, Manley G, Dalmau J and Posner J 1996. The HuD paraneoplastic protein shares immunogenic regions between PEM/PSN patients and several strains and species of experimental animals. *J. Neuroimmunol.* 71: 199-206.

Sommer C, Weishaupt A, Brinkhoff J, Biko L, Wessig C, Gold R and Toyka KV 2005. Paraneoplastic stiff-person syndrome: passive transfer to rats by means of IgG antibodies to amphiphysin. *Lancet.* 365: 1406-11.

Tanaka K, Ding X and Tanaka M 2004. Effects of antineuronal antibodies from patients with paraneoplastic neurological syndrome on primary-cultured neurons. *J. Neurol. Sci.* 217: 25-30.

Tanaka K, Tanaka M, Inuzuka T, Nakano R and Tsuji S 1999. Cytotoxic T lymphocyte-mediated cell death in paraneoplastic sensory neuronopathy with anti-Hu antibody. *J. Neurol. Sci.* 163: 159-62.

Tanaka M, Tanaka K, Onodera O and Tsuji S 1995. Trial to establish an animal model of paraneoplastic cerebellar degeneration with anti-Yo antibody. 1. Mouse strains bearing different MHC molecules produce antibodies on immunization with recombinant Yo protein, but do not cause Purkinje cell loss. *Clin. Neurol. Neurosurg.* 97: 95-100.

Tanaka M, Tanaka K, Shinozawa K, Idezuka J and Tsuji S 1998. Cytotoxic T cells react with recombinant Yo protein from a patient with paraneoplastic cerebellar degeneration and anti-Yo antibody. *J. Neurol. Sci.* 161: 88-90.

Thieben MJ, Lennon VA, Boeve BF, Aksamit AJ, Keegan M and Vernino S 2004. Potentially reversible autoimmune limbic encephalitis with neuronal potassium channel antibody. *Neurology.* 62: 1177-82.

Vincent A 2006. Immunology of disorders of neuromuscular transmission. *Acta Neurol. Scand. Suppl.* 183: 1-7.

Vincent A, Irani SR and Lang B 2010. The growing recognition of immunotherapy-responsive seizure disorders with autoantibodies to specific neuronal proteins. *Curr. Opin. Neurol.* 23: 144-50.

Voltz R, Dalmau J, Posner JB and Rosenfeld MR 1998. T-cell receptor analysis in anti-Hu associated paraneoplastic encephalomyelitis. *Neurology.* 51: 1146-50.

Yu Z, Kryzer TJ, Griesmann GE, Kim K, Benarroch EE and Lennon VA 2001. CRMP-5 neuronal autoantibody: marker of lung cancer and thymoma-related autoimmunity. *Ann. Neurol.* 49: 146-54.

Chapter 5

MOVEMENT DISORDERS

Ruth Huizinga[1] and Sandra Amor[2,3]
[1] Department of Immunology, Erasmus MC,
University Medical Center, Rotterdam, The Netherlands.
[2] Department of Pathology, VU Medical Center Amsterdam,
The Netherlands.
[3] Neuroscience and Trauma Centre,
Barts and the London School of Medicine and Dentistry,
Queen Mary University of London, United Kingdom.

INTRODUCTION

Movement disorders of the central nervous system include encephalitic lethargica, Sydenham's chorea, Parkinson's disease and PANDAS (pediatric autoimmune disorders associated with streptococcal infections). Some of these movement disorders are associated with antibodies to basal ganglia neurons and develop after infection with group A β-haemolytic streptococcal bacteria (Streptococcus pyogenes). As most autoantibodies in these disorders are directed against intracellular antigens, the evidence for a pathogenic role as determined in animal models is still scarce.

ENCEPHALITIS LETHAGICA

In 1916 von Economo described a neurological disease characterized by a sleep associated with basal ganglia signs and neuropsychiatric sequele. While there was speculation that Encephalitis lethargica (EL) was associated with the 1918 influenza pandemic, investigators found no evidence of influenza RNA (McCall *et al.*, 2001). More recently, a group of patients was described with similar characteristics as von Ecomos EL patients also developing sequele following pharyngitis (Dale *et al.*, 2004). Rather than viral aetiology, antibodies to streptolysin-O were elevated in 65% of the patients, suggesting that infection with Streptococcus could be a possible trigger for the disease. EL patients develop antibodies against cells within the basal ganglia and respond well to steroids suggesting a role for autoimmunity in disease in particular anti-basal ganglia (neuronal) antibodies (Church *et al.*, 2003). Recently, antibodies to the N-methyl-D-aspartate (NMDA) receptor, expressed on the cell membrane of many neurons, have been described in 50% of EL cases (Dale *et al.*, 2009).

SYDENHAM'S CHOREA

Sydenham's chorea, historically known as Saint Vitus' dance, is a neurological movement disorder characterised by involuntary purposeless movements, predominantly of the face, feet and hands. Motor weakness may develop in some cases as well (Dale, 2005). The disease typically occurs in children and is mostly transient with an average duration of nine months. Sydenham's chorea is a neurological complication of acute rheumatic fever which occurs after infection with group A β-haemolytic streptococcal bacteria. It can occur simultaneously with other complications of post-streptococcal infections such as rheumatic heart disease and arthritis.

Patients with Sydenham's chorea develop antibodies against cells within the basal ganglia (Church *et al.*, 2002, Husby *et al.*, 1976, Swedo *et al.*, 1993). These antibodies probably arise through a mechanism of molecular mimicry due to cross-reactivity with streptococcal infections (Kirvan *et al.*, 2003), although their pathogenicity remains unknown (Martino and Giovannoni, 2004). Serum from patients with Sydenham's chorea, but not other streptococcal disorders, bound to the surface of human neuronal cells and recognised the neuronal glycolytic enzymes aldolase C, γ-gamma-enolase, and pyruvate kinase (Dale *et al.*, 2006). In addition, tubulin has been identified as a target for the autoantibodies (Kirvan *et al.*, 2007). Subsequent studies showed that anti-basal ganglia antibodies were also present in other patients with post-streptococcal infection presenting with a spectrum of movement and psychiatric disorders. The association of the antibodies with the disease was further examined *in vitro* whereby serum from patients with Sydenham's chorea were found to induce calcium/calmodulin-dependent protein (CaM) kinase activity that leads to dopamine release (Kirvan *et al.*, 2006). While further studies are necessary to define the mode of action of antineuronal antibodies in Sydenham's chorea itself, it was demonstrated that commercial antibodies to neuronal glycolytic enzymes induced apoptosis in cultured neurons (Dale *et al.*, 2006).

PANDAS

PANDAS is an acronym for pediatric autoimmune disorders associated with streptococcal infections. Children with this syndrome show an acute onset of obsessive-compulsive behaviour, hyperreactivity, tics and emotional lability after infection with group A β-haemolytic streptococcus. MRI studies indicated a larger volume of the caudate, putamen and globus pallidus in these patients, suggesting that the basal ganglia dysfunction is underlying the neuropsychiatric symptoms (Giedd *et al.*, 2000). Both plasma exchange and treatment with intravenous immunoglobulin (IVIg) have beneficial effects suggesting that antibodies play a role in this disease, at least in a subset of patients (Perlmutter *et al.*, 1999). Similar to Sydenham's chorea, patients with PANDAS have antibodies reactive with basal ganglia antigens, although other studies have not found a higher prevalence of these antibodies as compared to healthy controls (Singer *et al.*, 2005). Antibodies cross-reactive with Streptococcus bacteria have been shown to bind lysoganglioside GM1, which is present on the surface of neuronal cells (Kirvan *et al.*, 2006).

PARKINSON'S DISEASE

Idiopathic Parkinson's disease (PD) is a progressive neurological disorder characterised by loss of motor control as observed by for example rigidity of muscles and gait dysfunction. The pathology of PD is predominantly the degeneration of dopaminergic (DA) neurons within the substantial nigra and intracytoplasmic inclusions known as Lewy bodies which contain accumulated alpha-synuclein fibrillar aggregates. The cause of PD is unknown although mutations in e.g. alpha-synuclein have been implicated in susceptibility to disease. While alpha-synuclein can form several different aggregate morphologies including oligomers, protofibrils and fibrils, the role of these morphologies in the progression of PD is not known.

It is clear that immune responses play a crucial role in disease since substantia nigra degeneration is associated with microglia activation and anti-inflammatory approaches appear to control disease. Gamma delta+ T cells are increased in patients with PD (Fiszer *et al.*, 1994) and more recently it was reported that immunoglobulin was present on DA neurons and Lewy bodies in PD patients while FcR were expressed by adjacent microglia (Orr *et al.*, 2005). Whether the elevated gamma delta+ T cell population in Parkinson's disease reflects previously unrecognized inflammation or may occur also in non-inflammatory disorders remains to be elucidated. The strongest evidence that autoimmunity to DA neurons may play a role in disease comes from studies showing that the CSF of patients is toxic to DA cells in culture (Dahlstrom *et al.*, 1990) via complement-dependent mechanisms (Defazio *et al.*, 1994). Furthermore microinjection of IgG from the sera of PD patients in the substantia nigra of rats induced severe neuronal loss concomitant with microglia activation. That microglia, activated by lipopolysaccharide, induced injury to dopaminergic neurons in cultures (Le *et al.*, 2001), suggests that activated microglia could also induce neurological disease in vivo. The role for Fcgamma receptors on microglia in the autoimmune attack on nigral neurones is reflected by the lack of neuronal damage in mice lacking Fcgamma receptors following injection of IgG from PD patients (He *et al.*, 2002). More recently (Huber *et al.*, 2006) showed that antibodies in the sera of PD patients bind to DA neurons and reduce dopamine production suggesting the potential for autoimmunity in disease. A subset of patients with PD have antibodies to aldolase C, neuron-specific enolase or pyruvate kinase and these antibodies correlated with the presence of atypical disease symptoms (van de Warrenburg *et al.*, 2008).

ANIMAL MODELS

The relevance of anti-brain antibodies in the movement disorder Tourette's syndrome was examined in rats infused with serum or purified IgG from patients. The antibodies induced involuntary movements in the animals similar to that seen in patients and examination of the CNS demonstrated antibodies bound to the striatal neurons (Hallett *et al.*, 2000). It remains to be determined if this observation occurs in other disorders or if there is a pathogenic role for cell mediated immune response to basal ganglia antigens. To establish a model of these disorders SJL/J mice were immunized with homogenates of the group A β-haemolytic streptococcal bacteria in CFA (Hoffman *et al.*, 2004). Mice developed behavioural changes and autoantibodies in the serum that reacted histologically against neurons within the deep cerebellar nuclei, globus pallidus, and thalamus. In addition IgG deposits were observed in the neurons suggesting that anti-streptococcal antibodies cross-reactive with brain components may play a role in disease.

To investigate a pathogenic role for autoimmune mechanisms in PD guinea pigs were immunized with homogenates of bovine mesencephalon (containing neurons of the substantia nigra). While no overt clinical signs of basal ganglia dysfunction were observed animals showed evidence of neuronal damage in the substantia nigra concomitant with a decrease in tyrosine hydroxylase activity and dopamine content. IgG was observed in neurons in the substantia nigra (Appel *et al.*, 1992). In a follow-up study, guinea pigs were immunized with dopaminergic MES 23.5 cells which resulted in hypokinesia in over 50% of the animals (Le *et al.*, 1995). Severe loss of substantia nigra neurons, decreased tyrosine hydroxylase activity and dopamine content as well as IgG deposition within neurons in the substantial nigra was observed. These data suggest that a similar mechanism in which autoimmunity to substantia nigra neurons induces neurodegeneration in animals may operate in Parkinson's disease in humans.

REFERENCES

Appel SH, Le WD, Tajti J, Haverkamp LJ and Engelhardt JI 1992. Nigral damage and dopaminergic hypofunction in mesencephalon-immunized guinea pigs. *Ann. Neurol.* 32: 494-501.

Church AJ, Cardoso F, Dale RC, Lees AJ, Thompson EJ and Giovannoni G 2002. Anti-basal ganglia antibodies in acute and persistent Sydenham's chorea. *Neurology.* 59: 227-31.

Church AJ, Dale RC, Cardoso F, Candler PM, Chapman MD, Allen ML, Klein NJ, Lees AJ and Giovannoni G 2003. CSF and serum immune parameters in Sydenham's chorea: evidence of an autoimmune syndrome? *J. Neuroimmunol.* 136: 149-53.

Dahlstrom A, Wigander A, Lundmark K, Gottfries CG, Carvey PM and McRae A 1990. Investigations on auto-antibodies in Alzheimer's and Parkinson's diseases, using defined neuronal cultures. *J. Neural. Transm. Suppl.* 29: 195-206.

Dale RC 2005. Post-streptococcal autoimmune disorders of the central nervous system. *Dev. Med. Child Neurol.* 47: 785-91.

Dale RC, Candler PM, Church AJ, Wait R, Pocock JM and Giovannoni G 2006. Neuronal surface glycolytic enzymes are autoantigen targets in post-streptococcal autoimmune CNS disease. *J. Neuroimmunol.* 172: 187-97.

Dale RC, Church AJ, Surtees RA, Lees AJ, Adcock JE, Harding B, Neville BG and Giovannoni G 2004. Encephalitis lethargica syndrome: 20 new cases and evidence of basal ganglia autoimmunity. *Brain.* 127: 21-33.

Dale RC, Irani SR, Brilot F, Pillai S, Webster R, Gill D, Lang B and Vincent A 2009. N-methyl-D-aspartate receptor antibodies in pediatric dyskinetic encephalitis lethargica. *Ann. Neurol.* 66: 704-9.

Defazio G, Dal Toso R, Benvegnu D, Minozzi MC, Cananzi AR and Leon A 1994. Parkinsonian serum carries complement-dependent toxicity for rat mesencephalic dopaminergic neurons in culture. *Brain Res.* 633: 206-12.

Fiszer U, Mix E, Fredrikson S, Kostulas V, Olsson T and Link H 1994. gamma delta+ T cells are increased in patients with Parkinson's disease. *J. Neurol. Sci.* 121: 39-45.

Giedd JN, Rapoport JL, Garvey MA, Perlmutter S and Swedo SE 2000. MRI assessment of children with obsessive-compulsive disorder or tics associated with streptococcal infection. *Am. J. Psychiatry.* 157: 281-3.

Hallett JJ, Harling-Berg CJ, Knopf PM, Stopa EG and Kiessling LS 2000. Anti-striatal antibodies in Tourette syndrome cause neuronal dysfunction. *J. Neuroimmunol.* 111: 195-202.

He Y, Le WD and Appel SH 2002. Role of Fcgamma receptors in nigral cell injury induced by Parkinson disease immunoglobulin injection into mouse substantia nigra. *Exp. Neurol.* 176: 322-7.

Hoffman KL, Hornig M, Yaddanapudi K, Jabado O and Lipkin WI 2004. A murine model for neuropsychiatric disorders associated with group A beta-hemolytic streptococcal infection. *J. Neurosci.* 24: 1780-91.

Huber VC, Mondal T, Factor SA, Seegal RF and Lawrence DA 2006. Serum antibodies from Parkinson's disease patients react with neuronal membrane proteins from a mouse dopaminergic cell line and affect its dopamine expression. *J. Neuroinflammation.* 3: 1.

Husby G, van de Rijn I, Zabriskie JB, Abdin ZH and Williams RC, Jr. 1976. Antibodies reacting with cytoplasm of subthalamic and caudate nuclei neurons in chorea and acute rheumatic fever. *J. Exp. Med.* 144: 1094-110.

Kirvan CA, Cox CJ, Swedo SE and Cunningham MW 2007. Tubulin is a neuronal target of autoantibodies in Sydenham's chorea. *J. Immunol.* 178: 7412-21.

Kirvan CA, Swedo SE, Heuser JS and Cunningham MW 2003. Mimicry and autoantibody-mediated neuronal cell signaling in Sydenham chorea. *Nat. Med.*9: 914-20.

Kirvan CA, Swedo SE, Kurahara D and Cunningham MW 2006. Streptococcal mimicry and antibody-mediated cell signaling in the pathogenesis of Sydenham's chorea. *Autoimmunity.* 39: 21-9.

Le W, Rowe D, Xie W, Ortiz I, He Y and Appel SH 2001. Microglial activation and dopaminergic cell injury: an in vitro model relevant to Parkinson's disease. *J. Neurosci.* 21: 8447-55.

Le WD, Engelhardt J, Xie WJ, Schneider L, Smith RG and Appel SH 1995. Experimental autoimmune nigral damage in guinea pigs. *J. Neuroimmunol.* 57: 45-53.

Martino D and Giovannoni G 2004. Antibasal ganglia antibodies and their relevance to movement disorders. *Curr. Opin. Neurol.*17: 425-32.

McCall S, Henry JM, Reid AH and Taubenberger JK 2001. Influenza RNA not detected in archival brain tissues from acute encephalitis lethargica cases or in postencephalitic Parkinson cases. *J. Neuropathol. Exp. Neurol.* 60: 696-704.

Orr CF, Rowe DB, Mizuno Y, Mori H and Halliday GM 2005. A possible role for humoral immunity in the pathogenesis of Parkinson's disease. *Brain.* 128: 2665-74.

Perlmutter SJ, Leitman SF, Garvey MA, Hamburger S, Feldman E, Leonard HL and Swedo SE 1999. Therapeutic plasma exchange and intravenous immunoglobulin for obsessive-compulsive disorder and tic disorders in childhood. *Lancet.* 354: 1153-8.

Singer HS, Hong JJ, Yoon DY and Williams PN 2005. Serum autoantibodies do not differentiate PANDAS and Tourette syndrome from controls. *Neurology.* 65: 1701-7.

Swedo SE, Leonard HL, Schapiro MB, Casey BJ, Mannheim GB, Lenane MC and Rettew DC 1993. Sydenham's chorea: physical and psychological symptoms of St Vitus dance. *Pediatrics.* 91: 706-13.

van de Warrenburg BP, Church AJ, Martino D, Candler PM, Bhatia KP, Giovannoni G and Quinn NP 2008. Antineuronal antibodies in Parkinson's disease. *Mov. Disord.* 23: 958-63.

Chapter 6

AMYOTROPHIC LATERAL SCLEROSIS AND ALZHEIMER'S DISEASE

Ruth Huizinga[1] and Sandra Amor[2,3]
[1] Department of Immunology, Erasmus MC,
University Medical Center, Rotterdam, The Netherlands.
[2] Department of Pathology, VU Medical Center Amsterdam,
The Netherlands.
[3] Neuroscience and Trauma Centre,
Barts and the London School of Medicine and Dentistry,
Queen Mary University of London, United Kingdom.

INTRODUCTION

The neurodegenerative diseases amyotrophic lateral sclerosis (ALS) and Alzheimer's disease (AD) have distinct clinical manifestation yet both involve degeneration of neurons in which there is evidence for the involvement of innate and adaptive immune responses. In particular activated microglia are found at site of damage in both ALS and AD. More recently studies describe T cells at the sites of spinal cord motor neuron injury in ALS and antibodies in the serum of ALS and AD patients recognise neuronal structures implicating the immune system in the disorders. Supporting this idea is the finding that the presence of T reg cells is beneficial in a mouse model of ALS. More recently several novel ideas have arisen suggesting a potential role for abnormally folded proteins in activation of the innate immune system. Here we discuss the evidence for the role of the innate and adaptive immune responses in these diseases that appear to be both instigators of the neurodegeneration as well as aid recovery.

AMYOTROPHIC LATERAL SCLEROSIS

Amyotrophic lateral sclerosis (ALS) is the most common form of motor neuron disease affecting adults. Commonly known as Lou Gehrig's disease ALS is a rapidly progressive disorders resulting in weakness and atrophy of limb musculature, slurred speech, difficulty in swallowing and death usually occurs within 4-6 years after onset. The cause of the disease is unknown and to date therapies do not halt the disease. Research on the mechanisms of neurodegeneration has focussed on oxidative stress, glutaminergic exocitotoxicity and aberrant protein aggregation, such as superoxide dismutase (SOD). While the mechanisms of disease are unclear there is the gradual awareness from both human and experiment studies that such mutated and aggregated proteins play a major role in activating immune responses although it is unclear whether such responses are the cause or consequence of neuronal damage.

ALS involves a progressive degeneration of the motor neurons in the CNS both in the spinal cord and the brain. Most cases are sporadic while approximately 5-10% is caused by an autosomal dominant mutation. While over 140 mutations are now identified, the mutated form of SOD-1 gene (G93A) in the mouse model is linked with only 20% of ALS cases in which a mutation in the CU/Zn superoxide dismutase 1 (SOD1) occurs. SOD1 is a crucial anti-oxidant enzyme which is thought to prevent abnormal function and folding of proteins however misfolded SOD1 in neurons is insufficient to cause ALS in experimental models and studies indicate that mutated, aggregated and oxidised forms of SOD1 leads to activation of local microglia that trigger neuroinflammation and disease.

The Immune Response in ALS

The suggestion that neuroinflammation contributes to ALS is reflected by the presence of the chemokines MCP-1 in the CSF and increased levels of markers of inflammation in the serum of ALS patients that correlate with severity of disease (Holmoy et al., 2006). For example in ALS patients levels of IL-17A in the serum are significantly increased while IL-17 positive CD8 T cells and mast cells and TNF alpha positive macrophages co-localize with neurons. In culture mutated SOD1 protein induces proinflammatory cytokines production in monocytes indicating a possible role for the mutated protein in the CNS (Fiala *et al.*, 2010).

Autoimmune Responses in ALS

Although ALS has also been suggested to be an unconventional autoimmune disease (Drachman and Kuncl, 1989) it is unclear whether such responses arise due to neuronal damage. The idea that the immune response maybe involved in ALS is supported by findings of autoimmunity to neuronal antigens since immunoglobulin is present in the motor neurons of ALS patients more frequently than serum from controls (Fishman and Drachman, 1995; Engelhardt *et al.*, 2005). IgG and IgM to spinal cord proteins and gangliosides (GM1 is located on the outer surface of motor neurons) are present in the serum and CSF of ALS patients (Annunziata *et al.*, 1995, Niebroj-Dobosz *et al.*, 2006, Niebroj-Dobosz *et al.*, 2004) and responses to NF associated with the slow evolution of disease in a subgroup of patients (Couratier *et al.*, 1998). In a more extensive study high frequency of antibodies to tubulin and NF-H were observed in ALS patients but also observed in patients with other neurological disorders (Terryberry *et al.*, 1998). In culture IgG from ALS patients recognises L-type VGCC resulting in an inhibition of dopamine mediated by L-type calcium channels in cultured PC12 cells (Offen *et al.*, 1998) and induces calcium dependent motor neuron cell death that is prevented by preincubating IgG with purified intact L-type VGCC (Smith *et al.*, 1994).

Animal Models of ALS

The most extensively used animal model of ALS is the mutant (m) SOD1 mouse. These mice develop ALS yet expression of mSOD1 in the neurons alone does not lead to ALS while ablating microglia expression of mSOD1 increases the lifespan of these mice. Such mice produce antibodies to the mutated protein although the disease is similar in B cell deficient mice suggesting that such reposes do not play a major role in the experimental model.

That ALS Ig may have a pathogenic effect in vivo was demonstrated following injection of mice with IgG from ALS patients. IgG form ALS patients (but not from people without ALS) was observed in motor neurons and at the neuromuscular junction of mice (Appel *et al.*, 1991). These mice had increased miniature end-plate potential frequency, with normal amplitude and time course and normal resting membrane potential, indicating an increased resting quantal release of acetylcholine from the nerve terminal. Similar studies were reported by Pullen and Humphreys (2000) in which Ig from ALS patients was present in the cell bodies of lumbar motor neurons and EM studies revealed histological abnormalities including abnormal formation of Nissle bodies and fragmented Golgi and ER.

Several models of ALS have been developed and have contributed to the understanding of ALS. For example the pathogenic role for autoimmune responses to neuronal antigens was demonstrated in guinea pigs immunised with purified bovine spinal motor neurons or with bovine spinal cord ventral horn homogenate (Engelhardt *et al.*, 1989, Engelhardt *et al.*, 1990). Immunisation with purified bovine spinal motor neurons caused signs of lower motor neuron deficits. In comparison guinea pigs immunised with bovine spinal cord ventral horn homogenate developed acute muscle weakness and paresis concomitant with inflammation in the CNS and both upper and lower motor neuron degeneration. As with the human disorder, IgG deposits at the motor end plate and within the motor neurons were observed. Passive transfer with immunoglobulin from guinea pigs with disease into naive mice demonstrated the presence of IgG in motor neurons and at the neuromuscular junction. Similar to the finding following injection of Ig from an ALS patient the mice showed an increase in miniature end-plate potential frequency providing evidence for autoimmune mechanisms in the pathogenesis of both the animal models and human ALS (Appel *et al.*, 1991). Immunisation of guinea pigs with choline acetyltransferase was shown to induce lower motoneuron destruction and striated muscle atrophy. As with the other models IgG was detected in lower motor neurons and at the motor end-plate and transfer of antibodies into mice induced selective lower motor neuron damage (Engelhardt *et al.*, 1997). While little is known about T cell responses in inducing neuronal damage T cells have been shown to be neuroprotective in an animal model of ALS (Chiu *et al.*, 2008).

ALZHEIMER'S DISEASE

Alzheimer's disease (AD) is the most common neurodegenerative disease leading to progressive cognitive decline and dementia. Clinically AD is characterised by the failure of memory and the gradual loss of acquired skills leading to apraxia, agnosia and aphasia. These clinical signs are the result of the neuropathological hallmarks of AD first described by Alois Alzheimer in 1907 (Alzheimer, 1907) that are thought to occur 20-30 years before manifestation of the clinical symptoms. Examination of the AD brain reveals neuronal loss and concomitant deposition of fibrils both extra cellular as well as within neurons. These deposits are most prevalent in the limbic system and the frontal, parietal and temporal cortex – all regions involved in memory and acquired skills.

While the extra-cellular deposits of fibrils mainly consist of amyloid β (Aβ) protein that arises from the proteolytic degradation of amyloid precursor protein (APP), the major component of the neurofibrillary tangles (NFTs) is hyperphosphorylated tau.

In the AD brain, such amyloid deposits containing fibrillar aggregates of Aβ protein are associated with activated microglia. Such activation is thought to aid removal of aggregated protein which while beneficial in early disease may eventually lead to chronic inflammation and neurological damage. More recent findings such suggest that, at least in the mouse model microglia activation does not play a role in removal of aggregated proteins although it remains to be seen whether the same is true in humans.

The conventional paradigm is that abnormally folded proteins accumulate in neurons leading to neuronal death via apoptosis. Alongside this idea is the accumulating evidence for a role of the immune response in the neuronal damage. As mentioned microglia activation leads to production of e.g. ROS in which neurons succumb to collateral damage. Therapeutic approaches also implicate the role of the immune system since epidemiological studies suggest that non-steroidal anti-inflammatory drugs (NSAIDs) can prevent or reduce the symptoms of Alzheimer's disease (AD) although clinical trials investigating the efficacy of NSAIDs in AD have proved inconclusive. One crucial fining is that autoantibodies against beta-amyloid that are common in Alzheimer's disease are thought to remove the aggregates and thus help control the disease (Kellner et al., 2009) although whether this eventually will translate to a therapy is unclear.

Immune Responses in AD

As discussed above several lines of evidence implicate the immune responses in the pathogenesis of AD and indeed have been targeted in approaches to remove aggregated proteins that contribute to neuro-degeneration. However, inflammatory processes, and possibly autoimmunity, may also play a role in disease since antibodies, complement components and T cells (CD4+ and CD8+) are observed in the brains of AD patients. Moreover, the presence of antibodies in sera of AD patients targeting specific neuronal antigens such as NF-H has lead to the suggestion that AD should be classified as an autoimmune disorder (D'Andrea, 2005) and autoantibodies have been used as biomarkers in disease (Colasanti *et al.*, 2010; Kim *et al.*, 2010) and correlate with cognitive impairment (Storace *et al.*, 2010). In an attempt to remove the accumulations of amyloid-β (Aβ) in the brains of AD patients, vaccinations with Aβ protein were unexpectedly resulting in severe meningoencephalitis, inflammation and worsening of the disease possibility due to autoimmune responses. Aβ is also recognised by T cells from AD patients although many reports are on antibody responses such as those directed to glial fibrillary protein (GFAP). In the search for autoantigens antibodies to spectrin (Fernandez-Shaw *et al.*, 1997), choline acetyltransferase (Engelhardt *et al.*, 1997), tau protein (Rosenmann *et al.*, 2006b) and aldolase A (Mor *et al.*, 2005) have been reported in AD. Autoimmunity to neuronal antigens is significantly higher in older (aged 70-79) than in younger (aged 40-59) subjects that may explain why neurodegenerative disorders generally occur at a later age. More specifically while the sera of older people recognised both bovine ventral root and dorsal root NF-H and their NF-H specificity was unchanged during aging the sera of AD patients contain IgG antibodies that bind more to ventral root cholinergic neurons which is enriched in phosphorylated NF-H, an observation that distinguished normal aged persons and those with AD (Soussan *et al.*, 1994). IgG responses to NF-H that binds specifically to epitopes highly enriched in Torpedo cholinergic neurons are also observed in older people with Down's syndrome that develop AD in later life (Hassin-Baer et al 1992).

Also in patients with AD antibodies to the extracellular domain of beta-amyloid precursor protein (APP) induced morphological changes in neuronal cultures consistent with apoptosis and may be the mechanism by which neuronal death in AD occurs (Rohn *et al.*, 2000). Of relevance to disease was the report that injection of purified IgG from AD patients into rat basal forebrain decreased the numbers of cholinergic neurons four weeks after injection of AD IgG. Injection of IgG from control patients had no effect, suggesting that autoimmunity may play a major role in neurodegeneration in AD patients (Engelhardt *et al.*, 2000).

Animal Models of AD

To examine the pathogenic potential of antibodies to cholinergic neurons Chapman *et al.* (1989) immunised rats with cholinergic neurons. Repeated immunizations induced antibody responses and immunoglobulin was detected in neurons and the animals displayed behavioural deficits involving spatial awareness and memory. In another study, Michaelson *et al.* (1990) also showed that repeated immunisation with cholinergic Torpedo neurons induced memory impairment in rats. Hippocampal neurons contained IgG and tangle-like structures. Experimental AD was also induced following prolonged immunisation of rats with NF-H protein of cholinergic neurons and again revealed IgG in neurons and cognitive deficits (Oron *et al.*, 1997) or immunisation of guinea pigs with septal cholinergic neurons (Kalman *et al.*, 1997).

Amyloid precursor protein (APP) and β-synuclein are neuronal proteins that accumulate in plaques in AD and PD. Immunisation with APP or β-synuclein was proposed as a therapy for reducing accumulation in the brain. Contrary to the expectations, some treated patients as well as mice immunised with APP peptide developed encephalitis (Furlan *et al.*, 2003, Nicoll *et al.*, 2003). Similarly, immunisation of rats with peptides of β-synuclein was shown to induce pathogenic T cells that resulted in acute paralytic encephalitis and uveitis following adoptive transfer (Mor *et al.*, 2003). In another study mice, immunised with recombinant human tau protein developed neurological deficits and histopathological features of AD and tauopathies, such as the presence of neurofibrillary tangle-like structures, axonal damage, gliosis and inflammation in the CNS (Rosenmann *et al.*, 2006a). Although the clinical signs of immunised mice do not mimic the symptoms observed in human AD, these data suggests that autoimmunity to neuronal antigens leads not only to neuronal deficits but also cognitive changes suggesting that autoimmunity may also play a role in human disease.

REFERENCES

Alzheimer A, Stelzmann RA, Schnitzlein HN and Murtagh FR 1995. An English translation of Alzheimer's 1907 paper, "Uber eine eigenartige Erkankung der Hirnrinde". *Clin. Anat.* 8: 429-31.

Annunziata P, Maimone D and Guazzi GC 1995. Association of polyclonal anti-GM1 IgM and anti-neurofilament antibodies with CSF oligoclonal bands in a young with amyotrophic lateral sclerosis. *Acta Neurol. Scand.* 92: 387-93.

Appel SH, Engelhardt JI, Garcia J and Stefani E 1991. Immunoglobulins from animal models of motor neuron disease and from human amyotrophic lateral sclerosis patients passively transfer physiological abnormalities to the neuromuscular junction. *Proc. Natl. Acad. Sci. U. S. A.* 88: 647-51.

Chapman J, Feldon J, Alroy G and Michaelson DM 1989. Immunization of rats with cholinergic neurons induces behavioral deficits. *J. Neural. Transplant.* 1: 63-76.

Chiu IM, Chen A, Zheng Y, Kosaras B, Tsiftsoglou SA, Vartanian TK, Brown RH, Jr. and Carroll MC 2008. T lymphocytes potentiate endogenous neuroprotective inflammation in a mouse model of ALS. *Proc. Natl. Acad. Sci. U. S. A.* 105: 17913-8.

Colasanti T, Barbati C, Rosano G, Malorni W and Ortona E 2010. Autoantibodies in patients with Alzheimer's disease: pathogenetic role and potential use as biomarkers of disease progression. *Autoimmun. Rev.* 9: 807-11.

Couratier P, Yi FH, Preud'homme JL, Clavelou P, White A, Sindou P, Vallat JM and Jauberteau MO 1998. Serum autoantibodies to neurofilament proteins in sporadic amyotrophic lateral sclerosis. *J. Neurol. Sci.* 154: 137-45.

D'Andrea MR 2005. Add Alzheimer's disease to the list of autoimmune diseases. *Med. Hypotheses.* 64: 458-63.

Drachman DB and Kuncl RW 1989. Amyotrophic lateral sclerosis: an unconventional autoimmune disease? *Ann. Neurol.* 26: 269-74.

Engelhardt JI, Appel SH and Killian JM 1989. Experimental autoimmune motoneuron disease. *Ann. Neurol.* 26: 368-76.

Engelhardt JI, Appel SH and Killian JM 1990. Motor neuron destruction in guinea pigs immunized with bovine spinal cord ventral horn homogenate: experimental autoimmune gray matter disease. *J. Neuroimmunol.* 27: 21-31.

Engelhardt JI, Le WD, Siklos L, Obal I, Boda K and Appel SH 2000. Stereotaxic injection of IgG from patients with Alzheimer disease initiates injury of cholinergic neurons of the basal forebrain. *Arch. Neurol.* 57: 681-6.

Engelhardt JI, Siklos L and Appel SH 1997. Immunization of guinea pigs with human choline acetyltransferase induces selective lower motoneuron destruction. *J. Neuroimmunol.* 78: 57-68.

Engelhardt JI, Soos J, Obal I, Vigh L and Siklos L 2005. Subcellular localization of IgG from the sera of ALS patients in the nervous system. *Acta Neurol. Scand.* 112: 126-33.

Fernandez-Shaw C, Marina A, Cazorla P, Valdivieso F and Vazquez J 1997. Anti-brain spectrin immunoreactivity in Alzheimer's disease: degradation of spectrin in an animal model of cholinergic degeneration. *J. Neuroimmunol.* 77: 91-8.

Fiala M, Chattopadhay M, La Cava A, Tse E, Liu G, Lourenco E, Eskin A, Liu PT, Magpantay L, Tse S, Mahanian M, Weitzman R, Tong J, Nguyen C, Cho T, Koo P, Sayre J, Martinez-Maza O, Rosenthal MJ and Wiedau-Pazos M 2010. IL-17A is increased in the serum and in spinal cord CD8 and mast cells of ALS patients. *J. Neuroinflammation.* 7: 76.

Fishman PS and Drachman DB 1995. Internalization of IgG in motoneurons of patients with ALS: selective or nonselective? *Neurology.* 45: 1551-4.

Furlan R, Brambilla E, Sanvito F, Roccatagliata L, Olivieri S, Bergami A, Pluchino S, Uccelli A, Comi G and Martino G 2003. Vaccination with amyloid-beta peptide induces autoimmune encephalomyelitis in C57/BL6 mice. *Brain.* 126: 285-91.

Hassin-Baer S, Wertman E, Raphael M, Stark V, Chapman J and Michaelson DM 1992. Antibodies from Down's syndrome patients bind to the same cholinergic neurofilament protein recognized by Alzheimer's disease antibodies. *Neurology.* 42: 551-5.

Holmoy T, Roos PM and Kvale EO 2006. ALS: cytokine profile in cerebrospinal fluid T-cell clones. *Amyotroph. Lateral Scler.* 7: 183-6.

Kalman J, Engelhardt JI, Le WD, Xie W, Kovacs I, Kasa P and Appel SH 1997. Experimental immune-mediated damage of septal cholinergic neurons. *J. Neuroimmunol.* 77: 63-74.

Kellner A, Matschke J, Bernreuther C, Moch H, Ferrer I and Glatzel M 2009. Autoantibodies against beta-amyloid are common in Alzheimer's disease and help control plaque burden. *Ann. Neurol.* 65: 24-31.

Kim I, Lee J, Hong HJ, Jung ES, Ku YH, Jeong IK, Cho YM, So I, Park KS and Mook-Jung I 2010. A relationship between Alzheimer's disease and type 2 diabetes mellitus through the measurement of serum amyloid-beta autoantibodies. *J. Alzheimers Dis.* 19: 1371-6.

Michaelson DM, Kadar T, Weiss Z, Chapman J and Feldon J 1990. Immunization with cholinergic cell bodies induces histopathological changes in rat brains. *Mol. Chem. Neuropathol.* 13: 71-80.

Mor F, Izak M and Cohen IR 2005. Identification of aldolase as a target antigen in Alzheimer's disease. *J. Immunol.* 175: 3439-45.

Mor F, Quintana F, Mimran A and Cohen IR 2003. Autoimmune encephalomyelitis and uveitis induced by T cell immunity to self beta-synuclein. *J. Immunol.* 170: 628-34.

Nicoll JA, Wilkinson D, Holmes C, Steart P, Markham H and Weller RO 2003. Neuropathology of human Alzheimer disease after immunization with amyloid-beta peptide: a case report. *Nat. Med.* 9: 448-52.

Niebroj-Dobosz I, Dziewulska D and Janik P 2006. Auto-antibodies against proteins of spinal cord cells in cerebrospinal fluid of patients with amyotrophic lateral sclerosis (ALS). *Folia Neuropathol.* 44: 191-6.

Niebroj-Dobosz I, Janik P and Kwiecinski H 2004. Serum IgM anti-GM1 ganglioside antibodies in lower motor neuron syndromes. *Eur. J. Neurol.* 11: 13-6.

Offen D, Halevi S, Orion D, Mosberg R, Stern-Goldberg H, Melamed E and Atlas D 1998. Antibodies from ALS patients inhibit dopamine release mediated by L-type calcium channels. *Neurology.* 51: 1100-3.

Oron L, Dubovik V, Novitsky L, Eilam D and Michaelson DM 1997. Animal model and in vitro studies of anti neurofilament antibodies mediated neurodegeneration in Alzheimer's disease. *J. Neural Transm. Suppl.* 49: 77-84.

Pullen AH and Humphreys P 2000. Ultrastructural analysis of spinal motoneurones from mice treated with IgG from ALS patients, healthy individuals, or disease controls. *J. Neurol. Sci.* 180: 35-45.

Rohn TT, Ivins KJ, Bahr BA, Cotman CW and Cribbs DH 2000. A monoclonal antibody to amyloid precursor protein induces neuronal apoptosis. *J. Neurochem.* 74: 2331-42.

Rosenmann H, Grigoriadis N, Karussis D, Boimel M, Touloumi O, Ovadia H and Abramsky O 2006a. Tauopathy-like abnormalities and neurologic deficits in mice immunized with neuronal tau protein. *Arch. Neurol.* 63: 1459-67.

Rosenmann H, Meiner Z, Geylis V, Abramsky O and Steinitz M 2006b. Detection of circulating antibodies against tau protein in its unphosphorylated and in its neurofibrillary tangles-related phosphorylated state in Alzheimer's disease and healthy subjects. *Neurosci. Lett.* 410: 90-3.

Smith RG, Alexianu ME, Crawford G, Nyormoi O, Stefani E and Appel SH 1994. Cytotoxicity of immunoglobulins from amyotrophic lateral sclerosis patients on a hybrid motoneuron cell line. *Proc. Natl. Acad. Sci. U. S. A.* 91: 3393-7.

Soussan L, Tchernakov K, Bachar-Lavi O, Yuvan T, Wertman E and Michaelson DM 1994. Antibodies to different isoforms of the heavy neurofilament protein (NF-H) in normal aging and Alzheimer's disease. *Mol. Neurobiol.* 9: 83-91.

Storace D, Cammarata S, Borghi R, Sanguineti R, Giliberto L, Piccini A, Pollero V, Novello C, Caltagirone C, Smith MA, Bossu P, Perry G, Odetti P and Tabaton M 2010. Elevation of {beta}-amyloid 1-42 autoantibodies in the blood of amnestic patients with mild cognitive impairment. *Arch. Neurol.* 67: 867-72.

Terryberry JW, Thor G and Peter JB 1998. Autoantibodies in neurodegenerative diseases: antigen-specific frequencies and intrathecal analysis. *Neurobiol. Aging.* 19: 205-16.

Chapter 7

OTHER NEUROLOGICAL DISORDERS

Ruth Huizinga[1] and Sandra Amor[2,3]
[1] Department of Immunology, Erasmus MC,
University Medical Center, Rotterdam, The Netherlands.
[2] Department of Pathology, VU Medical Center Amsterdam,
The Netherlands.
[3] Neuroscience and Trauma Centre,
Barts and the London School of Medicine and Dentistry,
Queen Mary University of London, United Kingdom.

INTRODUCTION

Immune responses to neurons and axons are frequently associated with the neurodegenerative disorders such as amyotrophic lateral sclerosis, Alzheimer's disease, paraneoplastic disorders and multiple sclerosis. Supporting the possible role of such responses in patients is the findings that in animals, experimentally induced autoimmunity to neurons and axons lead to neurodegenerative disorders.

Autoimmune responses to neuronal and axonal antigens are also observed in other neurological disorders although there is far less evidence for the exact role of such responses. Here we discuss the evidence and possible role of autoimmunity to neuronal antigens in psychiatric disorders, epilepsy, systemic lupus erythematosus, autism, brain trauma and infections of the nervous system.

PSYCHIATRIC DISORDERS

Growing evidence also demonstrates the presence of autoantibodies to neurons in psychiatric disorders such as schizophrenia (Margutti et al., 2006) and in autistic disorders in which patients display impaired socialisation and abnormal patterns of behaviour.

The autistic spectrum disorders are a spectrum of neuro-developmental disorders, the aetiology or aetiologies of which remain unknown. Increasing evidence of autoimmunity in autistic people may be the result of the presence of altered or inappropriate immune responses in this disorder, and this immune system dysfunction may represent novel targets for treatment. While the exact cause of these disorders is unknown, genetic, biochemical and environmental causes have been suggested to play a role. One factor may be abnormal immune responses since autism is frequently observed in families in which autoimmune disorders occur. Furthermore, studies also reveal the presence of antibodies to foetal brain tissues in some mothers of children with autism. In experimental models these antibodies alter behaviour indicating that the same is true in humans. In some autistic people autoantibodies to myelin proteins and neuronal antigens such as neurofilament (NF) have been observed (Cohly and Panja, 2005) as well as altered T cell functions and cytokine levels (Zimmerman et al., 2005). In an extensive study examining responses to human brain proteins serum antibodies in autistic subjects more frequently and intensely responded to antigens in caudate, putamen and prefrontal cortex as well as cerebella and cingulated gyrus antigens than aged matched controls (Singer et al., 2006).

In a recent study Gonzalez-Gronow and colleagues (2010) observed antibodies to the voltage-dependent anion channel (VDAC) and hexokinase-I, a VDAC protective ligand, in autistic children. That these antibodies may play a role in neuronal dysfunction was suggested from in vitro studies showing that the antibodies induce apoptosis of cultured human neuroblastoma cells.

EPILEPSY

The concept that autoimmunity to neuronal antigens may be involved in some cases of epilepsy and seizure disorders is gained increasing interest. In chapter 5 we describe the presence of antibodies to voltage-gated potassium channels, N-methyl-D-aspartate receptors and glutamic acid decarboxylase

(GAD) in people with limbic encephalitis. However antibodies and T cells to other neuronal antigens antibodies may also play a role in these diseases.

Rasmussen's syndrome (RS) is a rare slowly progressive neurological childhood illness characterized by frequent and severe seizures, loss of motor skills and speech and paralysis on one side of the body. The encephalitis observed is suggested to result from autoimmunity following CMV and EBV infection although this is still controversial. The idea that neuronal damage is due to autoimmunity is reflected by serum antibodies and T cell responses to anti-glutamate receptor (GluR3) receptors in RS patients (Takahashi *et al.*, 2005). The pathogenic effect of antibodies to glutamate receptors (GluR), implicated in epilepsy and Rasmussen's syndrome, is reflected by their association with the frequency of seizures. In addition, plasma exchange and IVIg and immunosuppressive therapies have been shown to be effective in controlling disease in some patients. In cultured neuronal cells, antibodies to GluR3 act as ligands for AMPA subtype of glutamate receptors and evoke glutamate-like ion currents (Twyman *et al.*, 1995) which may explain the clinical phenotype in humans. The pathogenic potential of the AMPA receptor subunit GluR3 in RE was reported by Levite and Hermelin (1999) who immunised four strains of mice with the Glu3RB peptide (aa 372-395). The mice developed antibodies and T cells to the peptide and behavioural abnormalities but not epilepsy. The murine antibodies bound to neurons in vitro and evoked GluR channel activity, mimicking the pathophysiological effects of excess of glutamate inducing neuronal death (Levite *et al.*, 1999). In another study rabbits immunised with peptides of the receptor developed anti-GluR3 antibodies that bound to neuronal cultures and induced apoptosis (Twyman *et al.*, 1995). More relevant was the finding that the rabbits exhibited recurrent episodes of seizures as well as inflammatory lesions in the CNS resembling human RE. Taken together, these studies demonstrate that antibodies to a specific peptide of the GluR can kill neurons by an excitotoxic mechanism, and induce clinical features resembling the human disease RE.

SYSTEMIC LUPUS ERYTHEMATOSUS

Systemic lupus erythematosus (SLE) is a multi-organ autoimmune disorder in which the CNS may be involved and in which a significant loss of central neurons may occur. In some cases SLE patients present with Parkinsonian-like deficits, changes to the basal ganglia and axonal dysfunction although the underlying mechanisms of such damage are unknown. Antibodies to double stranded DNA (dsDNA), present in the serum of SLE patients, are known to deposit in the kidney and skin contributing to disease. (DeGiorgio *et al.*, 2001) demonstrated that a subset of the dsDNA antibodies, present in the CSF and serum of SLE patients also recognised NR2A and NR2B subunits of the NMDA receptor and reduced the viability of brain cells which proliferate *in vitro* (Sakic *et al.*, 2005). Responses to microtubule-associated protein 2 (MAP-2), a cellular protein restricted to neurons and important in the control of the cytoskeleton, is also a common finding in neuropsychiatric systemic lupus erythematosus (Williams *et al.*, 2004). That intrathecally synthesized IgG autoantibodies in SLE patients with neuropyschiatric disorder patient may be pathogenic is demonstrated by the finding that CSF IgG of SLE patients reduces the viability of a neural stem cell line in vitro (Sakic *et al.*, 2005). In a further study, anti-NMDAR antibodies in serum and cerebrospinal fluid from SLE patients induced cognitive impairment in mice injected with LPS to compromise the BBB integrity. Mice also exhibited neuron damage and memory impairment. Moreover immunoglobulin eluted from the brains of SLE patients, bound to DNA and NMDAR and caused neuronal apoptosis in mouse brains. Despite these findings further studies are necessary to reveal the mechanism of autoimmunity to NMDAR in neuropsychiatric lupus and the approaches by which such patients may be treated (Kowal *et al.*, 2006).

Spontaneous development of lupus-like disease in the MRL/lpr mouse model has been invaluable to study mechanism underlying neuropsychiatric SLE. SLE in the MRL/lpr mouse is accompanied by impaired dopamine catabolism and degenerating axon terminals in the mesencephalon (Hikawa *et al.*, 1997). Mice show behavioural dysfunction similar with progression of SLE in humans. The neurodegeneration in MRL/lpr mice (Ballok, 2007) is associated with the cytotoxicity of the IgG fraction CSF on neurons (Sidor *et al.*, 2005) which was attenuated by the immunosuppressive drug cyclophosphamide (Ballok *et al.*, 2004). Although the specificity of the mediators in the CSF is unknown, it is probable that autoimmunity to neurons contributes to pathology in the MRL/lpr mouse.

In a subset of SLE patients antibodies to NR2A and NR2B subunits of the NMDA receptor are present. The effect of antibodies to NR2 was studied in BALB/C mice in which epinephrine was used to compromise the BBB. These mice show a decrease in neurons in the lateral amygdala and develop cognitive and emotional behaviour changes (Huerta *et al.*, 2006).

BRAIN TRAUMA

During injury of the nervous system for example as a result of mechanical stress, antigens may become exposed to the immune system and provoke an autoimmune response.

In general autoimmunity is considered harmful to the host but more recent studies suggest that such responses may be protective following brain trauma (Stein *et al.*, 2002). Despite massive release of brain antigens as a result of trauma, and early expansion of myelin specific T cells in local lymph nodes, animals do not develop autoimmune neurological disease (Kwidzinski *et al.*, 2003). Brain trauma typically leads to neuronal damage and loss and while T cells reactive against myelin antigens are observed in 40% patients with traumatic brain injury (Cox *et al.*, 2006) few studies have examined the impact of anti-neuronal responses. Furthermore little is known about the impact of autoantibodies to neuronal antigens following brain trauma despite increased levels of NF-L in the CSF following cerebrovascular accidents, subacute haemorrhage and severe brain traumas (Van Geel *et al.*, 2005). While these may reflect the degree of axonal damage these antigens may also trigger a pathogenic immune response.

Shortly after brain trauma in humans IgG and IgM antibodies to β-tubulin class III (βTcIII), which is almost exclusively found in neuronal cytoskeletons is present in the serum (Skoda *et al.*, 2006). That these responses may be involved in the diseases is suggested by mouse studies (Ankeny *et al.*, 2006). To investigate the relevance of autoantibodies in patients with brain trauma serum from blood draining the CNS or systemic blood was applied to human leukaemia cell lines and apoptosis assessed with annexin V and propidium iodide staining. Serum draining the brain lesions and less so from systemic blood, induced cell death in vitro (Lopez-Escribano *et al.*, 2002).

The effect of autoimmunity generated in humans following brain trauma to neuronal cells is unknown and so far has only been studied in experimental models of brain trauma. More research is required to fully determine the pathogenic role of autoimmune responses in patients with brain trauma.

Extensive literature on brain injury is available in the many animal models of traumatic brain injury (Duhaime, 2006, Morales *et al.*, 2005). In adult rats in which brain trauma was induced, circulating IgG autoantibodies were also observed in degenerating neurons suggesting that anti-brain antibodies may be epiphenomenal (Rudehill *et al.*, 2006) or play a role in the phagocytosis and removal of injured neurons (Stein *et al.*, 2002). Alternatively such responses may contribute to axonal damage following prolonged exposure of the CNS to protein extravasation in severe fluid percussion injury in the rat brain (Hoshino *et al.*, 1996). In experimental spinal cord injury organ-specific and systemic autoimmune response is observed in mice and sera from the mice recognise CNS proteins and bind to DNA and RNA (Ankeny *et al.*, 2006). These data indicate that trauma to the CNS does evoke autoimmunity to CNS components and could induce disease although the evidence is weighted to such responses having a protective effect.

In contrast a recent report reveals that spinal cord injury (SCI) is less severe in mice lacking B cells (Ankeny *et al.*, 2009). Here these authors show that B cell sufficient mice develop severe disease with complement and Ig deposits at the site of the lesion correlating with axonal and myelin damage. In B cell deficient mice the pathology was dramatically reduced and locomotor recovery improved indicting that indeed antibodies to neuronal components could be pathogenic.

INFECTIONS

In spongiform encephalopathy neurofibrillary tangles similar to those observed in AD are observed particularly in Guamanians with Parkinson's disease. Scrapie associated fibrils of Kuru and CJD and has been suggested to be related to changes in ALS (Gajdusek, 1985). In all these diseases antibodies to neurofilaments are present and may have a common origin.

Autoimmunity to the neuronal antigen heterogeneous nuclear ribonuclear protein – A1 (hnRNP-A1) has been demonstrated in patients with human T-lymphotropic virus type 1 (HTLV-1) associated tropical spastic paraparesis (HAM/TSP). IgG isolated from HAM/TSP patients contains antibodies to neurons as determined by western blot studies on neuronal homogenates and more specifically to proteins identified as hnRNP-A1. A functional significance of such IgG in patients was confirmed using patch clamp recording of neurons from rat brain sections where infusion of IgG inhibited neuronal firing (Levin *et al.*, 2002).

REFERENCES

Ankeny DP, Lucin KM, Sanders VM, McGaughy VM and Popovich PG 2006. Spinal cord injury triggers systemic autoimmunity: evidence for chronic B lymphocyte activation and lupus-like autoantibody synthesis. *J. Neurochem.* 99: 1073-87.

Ankeny DP, Guan Z, Popovich PG. B cells produce pathogenic antibodies and impair recovery after spinal cord injury in mice. Clin Invest. 2009 Oct;119(10):2990-9. doi: 10.1172/JCI39780. Epub 2009 Sep 21.Ballok DA 2007. Neuroimmunopathology in a murine model of neuropsychiatric lupus. *Brain Res. Rev.* 54: 67-79.

Ballok DA, Earls AM, Krasnik C, Hoffman SA and Sakic B 2004. Autoimmune-induced damage of the midbrain dopaminergic system in lupus-prone mice. *J. Neuroimmunol.* 152: 83-97.

Cohly HH and Panja A 2005. Immunological findings in autism. *Int. Rev. Neurobiol.* 71: 317-41.

Cox AL, Coles AJ, Nortje J, Bradley PG, Chatfield DA, Thompson SJ and Menon DK 2006. An investigation of auto-reactivity after head injury. *J. Neuroimmunol.* 174: 180-6.

DeGiorgio LA, Konstantinov KN, Lee SC, Hardin JA, Volpe BT and Diamond B 2001. A subset of lupus anti-DNA antibodies cross-reacts with the NR2 glutamate receptor in systemic lupus erythematosus. *Nat. Med.* 7: 1189-93.

Duhaime AC 2006. Large animal models of traumatic injury to the immature brain. *Dev. Neurosci.* 28: 380-7.

Gonzalez-Gronow M, Cuchacovich M, Francos R, Cuchacovich S, Fernandez Mdel P, Blanco A, Bowers EV, Kaczowka S, Pizzo SV.Antibodies against the voltage-dependent anion channel (VDAC) and its protective ligand hexokinase-I in children with autism. *J. Neuroimmunol.* 2010 Oct 8;227(1-2):153-61.

Hikawa N, Kiuchi Y, Maruyama T and Takenaka T 1997. Delayed neurite regeneration and its improvement by nerve growth factor (NGF) in dorsal root ganglia from MRL-lpr/lpr mice in vitro. *J. Neurol. Sci.* 149: 13-7.

Hoshino S, Kobayashi S and Nakazawa S 1996. Prolonged and extensive IgG immunoreactivity after severe fluid-percussion injury in rat brain. *Brain. Res* 711: 73-83.

Huerta PT, Kowal C, DeGiorgio LA, Volpe BT and Diamond B 2006. Immunity and behavior: antibodies alter emotion. *Proc. Natl. Acad. Sci. U. S. A.* 103: 678-83.

Kowal C, Degiorgio LA, Lee JY, Edgar MA, Huerta PT, Volpe BT and Diamond B 2006. Human lupus autoantibodies against NMDA receptors mediate cognitive impairment. *Proc. Natl. Acad. Sci. U. S. A.* 103: 19854-9.

Kwidzinski E, Mutlu LK, Kovac AD, Bunse J, Goldmann J, Mahlo J, Aktas O, Zipp F, Kamradt T, Nitsch R and Bechmann I 2003. Self-tolerance in the immune privileged CNS: lessons from the entorhinal cortex lesion model. *J. Neural. Transm. Suppl.* 29-49.

Levite M, Fleidervish IA, Schwarz A, Pelled D and Futerman AH 1999. Autoantibodies to the glutamate receptor kill neurons via activation of the receptor ion channel. *J. Autoimmun.* 13: 61-72.

Levite M and Hermelin A 1999. Autoimmunity to the glutamate receptor in mice--a model for Rasmussen's encephalitis? *J. Autoimmun.* 13: 73-82.

Margutti P, Delunardo F and Ortona E 2006. Autoantibodies associated with psychiatric disorders. *Curr. Neurovasc. Res.* 3: 149-57.

Morales DM, Marklund N, Lebold D, Thompson HJ, Pitkanen A, Maxwell WL, Longhi L, Laurer H, Maegele M, Neugebauer E, Graham DI, Stocchetti N and McIntosh TK 2005. Experimental models of traumatic brain injury: do we really need to build a better mousetrap? *Neuroscience.* 136: 971-89.

Rudehill S, Muhallab S, Wennersten A, von Gertten C, Al Nimer F, Sandberg-Nordqvist AC, Holmin S and Mathiesen T 2006. Autoreactive antibodies against neurons and basal lamina found in serum following experimental brain contusion in rats. *Acta Neurochir. (Wien)* 148: 199-205; discussion 205.

Sakic B, Kirkham DL, Ballok DA, Mwanjewe J, Fearon IM, Macri J, Yu G, Sidor MM, Denburg JA, Szechtman H, Lau J, Ball AK and Doering LC 2005. Proliferating brain cells are a target of neurotoxic CSF in systemic autoimmune disease. *J. Neuroimmunol.* 169: 68-85.

Sidor MM, Sakic B, Malinowski PM, Ballok DA, Oleschuk CJ and Macri J 2005. Elevated immunoglobulin levels in the cerebrospinal fluid from lupus-prone mice. *J. Neuroimmunol.* 165: 104-13.

Singer HS, Morris CM, Williams PN, Yoon DY, Hong JJ and Zimmerman AW 2006. Antibrain antibodies in children with autism and their unaffected siblings. *J. Neuroimmunol.* 178: 149-55.

Skoda D, Kranda K, Bojar M, Glosova L, Baurle J, Kenney J, Romportl D, Pelichovska M and Cvachovec K 2006. Antibody formation against beta-tubulin class III in response to brain trauma. *Brain Res. Bull.* 68: 213-6.

Stagg CJ, Lang B, Best JG, McKnight K, Cavey A, Johansen-Berg H, Vincent A, Palace J. Autoantibodies to glutamic acid *Epilepsia.* 2010 Jun 7.

Stein TD, Fedynyshyn JP and Kalil RE 2002. Circulating autoantibodies recognize and bind dying neurons following injury to the brain. *J. Neuropathol. Exp. Neurol.* 61: 1100-8.

Takahashi Y, Mori H, Mishina M, Watanabe M, Kondo N, Shimomura J, Kubota Y, Matsuda K, Fukushima K, Shiroma N, Akasaka N, Nishida H, Imamura A, Watanabe H, Sugiyama N, Ikezawa M and Fujiwara T 2005. Autoantibodies and cell-mediated autoimmunity to NMDA-type GluRepsilon2 in patients with Rasmussen's encephalitis and chronic progressive epilepsia partialis continua. *Epilepsia.* 46 Suppl 5: 152-8.

Twyman RE, Gahring LC, Spiess J and Rogers SW 1995. Glutamate receptor antibodies activate a subset of receptors and reveal an agonist binding site. *Neuron.* 14: 755-62.

Van Geel WJ, Rosengren LE and Verbeek MM 2005. An enzyme immunoassay to quantify neurofilament light chain in cerebrospinal fluid. *J. Immunol. Methods.* 296: 179-85.

Vincent A, Irani SR, Lang B. The growing recognition *Curr. Opin. Neurol.* 2010 Apr;23(2):144-50. Review.

Williams RC, Jr., Sugiura K and Tan EM 2004. Antibodies to microtubule-associated protein 2 in patients with neuropsychiatric systemic lupus erythematosus. *Arthritis Rheum.* 50: 1239-47.

Zimmerman AW, Jyonouchi H, Comi AM, Connors SL, Milstien S, Varsou A and Heyes MP 2005. Cerebrospinal fluid and serum markers of inflammation in autism. *Pediatr. Neurol.* 33: 195-201.

Chapter 8

AUTOIMMUNITY TO NEURONAL ANTIGENS IN MULTIPLE SCLEROSIS

Baukje van der Star[1], Ruth Huizinga[2], Wouter Gerritsen[1] and Sandra Amor[1,3]

[1] Department of Pathology,
VU Medical Center Amsterdam, The Netherlands.
[2] Department of Immunology, Erasmus MC,
University Medical Center, Rotterdam, The Netherlands.
[3] Neuroscience and Trauma Centre,
Barts and the London School of Medicine and Dentistry,
Queen Mary University of London, United Kingdom.

ABSTRACT

Axonal damage is considered as the major cause of chronic disability in MS but the underlying pathological mechanisms are poorly understood. Similar to immune-mediated myelin destruction, autoimmunity to neuronal/axonal antigens may play an important role in axonal damage. T cell responses to neuronal antigens are observed in MS as well as in healthy controls indicating that such responses are part of the immune repertoire. Whether specific differences between responses in MS and controls differ is not known. Likewise, antibodies to neuronal and axonal antigens are observed in a range of diseases and healthy controls although higher responses correlate with the degree of neurodegeneration. That such antibodies play a role in disease comes from animal studies. Anti-axonal antibodies are pathogenic in animals and induce axonal damage. To model spasticity as observed in MS, immunisation of animals with neuronal antigens has been shown to induces neuronal and axonal damage and grey matter lesions along with clinical signs of neurological degeneration. Furthermore, immunoglobulin deposits are observed inside neurons and axons in these animals. Clearly auto-autoimmunity to axonal antigens plays an important role in mediating the axonal damage in animals indicting that such responses in MS may also be pathogenic merely than acting as a surrogate marker for axonal degeneration.

INTRODUCTION

Multiple Sclerosis (MS) is an immune-mediated neurodegenerative disease of the central nervous system (CNS). Pathologically the disease is characterised by demyelination and axonal loss associated with inflammation in which activated microglia and macrophages dominate the infiltrates (Rindfleisch, 1863, Charcot, 1868, Esiri and Reading, 1987). While research in MS has focussed on pathogenic T cells targeting myelin antigens relatively few studies have described the role for pathogenic antibodies to myelin antigens or indeed other CNS antigens such as neuronal proteins. Moreover despite Charcot's detailed description of the pathology of MS in a lecture in 1868 on the extent of inflammation and axon loss (Charcot, 1868), it has only been recently that researchers have returned to examine the mechanism of axonal damage and neuronal loss in MS. Undoubtedly the development of magnetic resonance spectroscopy (MRS) has allowed an unique view of the progression of the disease in patients. Such approaches have helped clarify the relationship of axonal damage and atrophy of the brain to the irreversible neurological disability. Nevertheless the cause of axonal damage remains unclear. As explained in previous chapters the role for autoimmunity, in particular auto-antibodies to neuronal antigens has been clearly demonstrated in several neurodegenerative disorders. The realisation that MS may also be classified as a neurodegenerative disorder in which auto-antibodies to neuronal antigens might play a role may help to not only uncover the pathogenic role for such autoimmune responses but may also lead to novel therapeutic strategies. The question now is whether there is any evidence for the involvement of autoimmunity to neuronal antigens in CNS disorders such as MS.

In MS several concepts have suggested how autoimmunity to myelin antigens may arise. One example is the presence of structures on viruses that are similar to myelin antigens – so called molecular mimicry (Fujinami and Oldstone, 1985). Yet another idea suggests that the progression of neurological disease is due to the phenomenon of determinant spreading (Lehmann *et al.,* 1993, Miller *et al.,* 1995). In this view the repertoire of the anti-myelin T cell responses that drives the disease becomes increasing dynamic with the generation of new reactivity's recognising antigens released with each new wave of disease. With these ideas in mind we discuss how autoimmunity to neuronal antigens may arise and, rather than to focus on the role of pathogenic T cells as is common in MS, we will discuss the evidence for auto-antibodies to neuronal antigens in MS. Understanding the mechanisms by which autoimmunity to neuronal antigens leads to neuronal injury is key to the development of effective therapies to prevent progression of disease and irreversible damage.

AXONAL DAMAGE AND NEURODEGENERATION IN MS

Studies from post-mortem spinal cord tissue from paralyzed MS patients has revealed that axonal damage correlates with irreversible neurological disability in paralyzed MS patients (Bjartmar *et al.,* 2000) indicating that control or arrest of progressive degeneration would be a crucial step in controlling disease progression. Although the extent of axonal injury is variable within and between lesions of MS patients, it is clearly present in all demyelinated lesions. In chronic active lesions there is severe axonal loss probably due to the extensive microglia activation (Figure 1A) and in chronic inactive lesions axonal density can be reduced up to 70% (Mews *et al.,* 1998, Bjartmar *et al.,* 2000). This may suggest that axonal injury occurs as a bystander effect to demyelination, however it is not restricted to the lesions. For example Kutzelnigg *et al.* (2005) observed axonal damage in the normal appearing white matter (NAWM), although such damage was observed less than that in chronic lesions. Interestingly Bitsch *et al.* (2000) suggested that axonal injury partially occurs independently of demyelination. They have based this hypothesis on the lack of correlation between axonal injury as measured by the amyloid-precursor protein (APP) expression and tumor necrosis factor-α (TNF-α) and inducible nitric oxide synthase (iNOS) mRNA expression in MS biopsy tissue. TNF-α and iNOS are both candidate mediators of demyelination (Selmaj and Raine, 1988, Mitrovic *et al.,* 1994). They do however observe a significant correlation between APP-positive axons and MHC-class II or CD8 positive T cells. More studies support the hypothesis of Bitsch and colleagues. For instance, a study performed by Bergers *et al* in 2002 shows that for a large part axonal damage does not correlate with signal abnormalities in the spinal cord measured by T2-weighted MRI.

For long it was thought that in MS, lesions only occurred in the normal appearing white matter. But with the improvement of magnetic resonance imaging (MRI) and histochemical staining techniques, it has become clear that demyelination and axonal degeneration can also occur in cortical regions (Kidd *et al.*, 1999). Also, grey matter pathology can be observed throughout the central nervous system. Since 1999 a classification system for grey matter (GM) lesions is used. Type I cortical lesions are localized both in white and grey matter. Type II cortical lesions are limited within the cortex (Figure 1B), so subcortical white matter and the surface of the cortex are not involved. Type III cortical lesions only include superficial layers of the cortex (subpial lesions) and finally type IV cortical lesions affect the subcortical regions (Kidd *et al.*, 1999, Bö *et al.*, 2006). Interestingly, in grey matter lesions infiltration of macrophages and lymphocytes is lower compared to white matter lesions (Bö *et al.*, 2003) and can sometimes be observed as a very clear border between the white and grey matter.

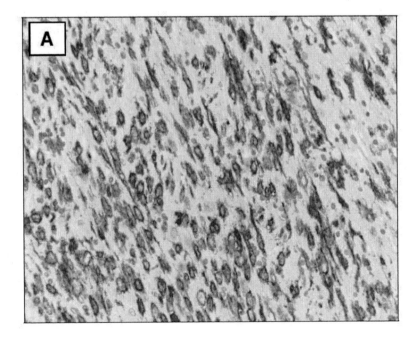

Figure 1 A. Extensive microglia activation in a chronic MS lesion. MHCII staining.

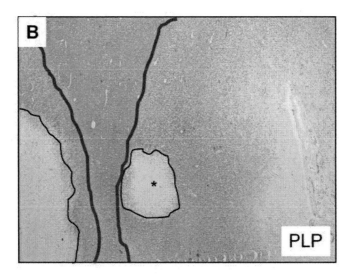

Figure 1B. Myelin loss in the grey matter. The white matter (between blue lines) in this tissue is unaffected. However myelin loss as depicted by lack of staining is clearly visible in the grey matter. A type II intracortical lesion (*) is circumscribed.

Although there seems to be no correlation between the location and the development of MS lesions (Ciccarelli *et al.,* 1999), there are however regions of the central nervous system that seem to be more vulnerable for the development of damage. These include the regions close to the ventricles (referred to as subventricular regions) and the optic nerve. There also seems to be a difference in vulnerability in neurons in the various levels in the spinal cord. For example, it has been shown that both motor- and interneurons were reduced in MS patients at the upper cervical and -thoracic level. However, this reduction was not observed in motor- and interneurons at the lumbar level (Gilmore *et al.,* 2009).

PROPOSED MECHANISMS OF AXONAL DAMAGE IN MS

Although the pathological mechanism of axonal injury is unknown, there have been several reports indicating a strong correlation with the degree of inflammation (Bitsch *et al.,* 2000, Fischer *et al.,* 2009). Besides, several studies have shown that inflammatory cells can contribute to axonal injury through the release of toxic factors. For example, the expression of iNOS is increased in acute MS lesions (Bö *et al.,* 1994, Liu *et al.,* 2001), what could lead to neurotoxic levels of nitric oxide (NO). NO can inhibit mitochondrial function causing reduced ATP production (Brorson *et al.*, 1999). Also an imbalanced glutamate homeostasis, reflected by an increased glutamate production, might contribute to axonal injury (Werner *et al.*, 2000, 2001). Amor and colleagues have reviewed the role of inflammation in neurodegeneration including the role of viral infections and the complement system in humans and animals (Amor *et al.*, 2010). Another proposed mechanism for the cause of axonal injury might be autoimmunity to neuronal proteins, or more specifically, axonal proteins. Next, we will discuss the evidence of this proposed mechanism in multiple sclerosis.

AUTOIMMUNITY TO NEURONAL/AXONAL ANTIGENS

In MS, both the innate and adaptive immune response are activated leading to an array of cells and molecules with either pro- or anti-inflammatory (or maybe both) effecter functions. Whereas in the innate immune response the dendritic cells, macrophages and neutral killer (NK) cells play a major role in killing bacteria-containing cells or parasites, in the adaptive immune response T and B lymphocytes are the effecter cells, stimulated by antigen presenting cells and their secreted factors. But it seems to be that both mechanisms are involved in MS, since macrophages, NK cells and T cells can be detected in MS lesions (Rindfleisch, 1863, Frommann, 1878, Traugott *et al.*, 1983, Newcombe *et al.*, 1994, Ulvestad *et al.*, 1994, Brück *et al.*, 1995). As well as activation of the innate immune response the adaptive immune response and specifically autoimmune responses could also play a specific role. Evidence for a role for autoimmunity against neuronal antigens is supported by several findings of axon reactive T and B lymphocytes in the cerebrospinal fluid (CSF) of patients with MS. For example Zhang *et al.* (2005a) isolated axon-reactive B-cells from the CSF of MS patients as well as detecting axon-reactive B cells and immunoglobulin (Ig) on axons in MS lesions (2005b). In a further study it was shown that the B-cells recognised the glycolytic enzymes triosephosphate isomerase (TPI) and glyceraldehyde-3-phosphate dehydrogenase (GAPDH) (Kolln *et al.*, 2006). Besides B lymphocytes also their effecter molecules, immunoglobulins, can be detected in MS lesions and are known as oligoclonal bands (OCBs) (Andersson *et al.*, 1994). However, not much is known about these Ig bands. For example, it is unknown what the targets of these immunoglobulins are and what the exact contribution to the disease is. Also, there seems to be no correlation between the presence and number of these OCBs in comparison with the disease course of relapsing-remitting MS (Koch *et al.*, 2007). Responses to neuraxonal proteins have also been observed by auto-reactive T cells, including responses to the neuron specific proteins enolase, arrestin (Forooghian *et al.*, 2007) and the neurofilament light subunit (NF-L) (Huizinga *et al.*, 2009). In the latter study, the proliferative responses of T lymphocytes to NF-L and MOG (myelin oligodendrocyte glycoprotein) were analysed using thymidine incorporation in peripheral blood mononuclear cells of MS patients and control subjects. The authors analysed the response of the different subtypes of T cells using fluorescent activated cell sorter (FACS) and detected a comparable response of CD3+CD4+ and CD3+CD8+ T cells after stimulation with NF-L. The presence of MOG induced a response dominated by CD3+CD4+ T. Since these responses were also present in healthy controls, this may indicate that these cells are part of the normal immune repertoire, suggesting the "need" for additional factors or components causing the T cell responses in MS to be autoreactive. Auto-antibodies could fill the gap in this mechanism.

Recognition of neurons and thus T cell activation leading to neurological damage requires the expression of key molecules for antigen presentation, such as major histocompatibility complex (MHC) and co-stimulatory molecules. The MHC-class I molecules are expressed on every cell membrane in the body, including neurons, and can be recognized solely by CD8 positive cytotoxic T cells. Whereas MHC-class II molecules are only expressed on the cell membrane of antigen presenting cells (APCs), including macrophages, microglia and dendritic cells, and can be recognized by CD4 positive T lymphocytes. Although it has become clear that CD8$^+$ T cells outnumber CD4+ T cells in MS lesions (Traugott *et al.*, 1983, Hauser *et al.*, 1986), very little information is available to show whether or how T cells may kill neurons. In the normal brain, neurons express negligible levels of MHC-class I probably to avoid such lethal consequences. However during inflammation neurons and axons may up regulate MHC-class I (Neumann *et al.*, 1995; Redwine *et al.*, 2001). Correspondingly, in MS lesions axons have been found positive for MHC-class I (Hoftberger *et al.*, 2004). Recently, Fissolo *et al.* (2009) have purified MHC-class I and MHC-class II molecules from brain autopsy samples from MS patients and analysed the eluted peptides from these molecules using mass spectrometry. Interestingly, NF-L, NF-M and α-synuclein peptides were found in this analysis. This suggests that through HLA-class I and class II molecules T cells can become activated and pathogenic directed to neuronal components resulting in neurodegeneration. *In vitro*, it has been shown that axons upregulate MHC-class I after IFN-γ and tetrodotoxin treatment, resulting in transection of neurites by cytotoxic T cells (Medana *et al.,* 2001). More evidence for the impact of T cells on neurons comes from studying interactions of PLP-specific T cells in brain slice cultures. While not specific for neurons, activated PLP-specific T cells induced calcium changes in neurons leading to neuronal damage (Nitsch *et al.,* 2004). Likewise MBP-specific T cells are more effective in activating microglia that have axon-damaging ability as observed in organotypic CNS cultures (Gimsa *et al.,* 2000) suggesting that in some way CNS specific T cells augment the CNS damage. Since T cell activation requires antigen presentation by APCs, the mechanisms leading to axonal injury may involve direct autoimmune-mediated damage (DeVries, 2004). This hypothesis can be supported by the detection of several auto-antibodies in the CSF and serum of MS patients. Mathey *et al.* (2007) showed that antibodies to a neuronal protein expressed at the Node of Ranvier, neurofascin-155/186 in serum of MS patients. Also antibodies directed to NF-L (Newcombe *et al.,* 1985, Terryberry *et al.,* 1998, Bartos *et al.,* 2007a), neurofilament medium (NF-M) (Bartos *et al.,* 2007b) and tubulin (Svarcová *et al.,* 2008) have been detected in the serum and CSF of MS patients. Among all subgroups in MS, patients with progressive disease seem to have elevated levels of antibodies to NF-L. In one study, patients with primary progressive MS had higher levels of antibodies to NF-L in the serum, but not in the CSF, than patients with secondary progressive MS (Ehling *et al.,* 2004). In another study, patients with primary progressive or secondary progressive MS had higher levels of antibodies to NF-L than patients with relapsing remitting MS (Silber *et al.,* 2002). These data might indicate that anti-neuronal immune responses may be important in a subset of MS patients. Significant differences in levels of NF-L antibodies between different MS subtypes, however, have not been found in other studies (Eikelenboom *et al.,* 2003), possibly due to differences in the selection of patients.

An important question is whether the antibody levels to neuroaxonal protein such as NF-L in MS patients are reflecting disease progression. To address this, anti-NF-L indices have been correlated with MRI measures of tissue damage. It appears that the anti-NF-L index in MS patients, especially in the relapsing remitting subgroup, correlates with MRI measures for axonal loss (Eikelenboom *et al.,* 2003). However, in that study there were no adjustments made for possible confounding factors, such as age which is known to influence both NF-L antibody levels and cerebral atrophy (Ehling *et al.,* 2004, Resnick *et al.,* 2003). NF-L, among other neuronal antigens, was also identified as an antigenic protein in MS, using serological proteome analysis. i.e. 2D SDS-PAGE, followed by immunoblotting and mass spectrometry (Almeras *et al.*, 2004). In another paper from that same group, NF-L was identified as a discriminate antigen between MS and healthy controls or Sjögren syndrome patients (Lefranc *et al.*, 2004). This study showed that the frequency of sera positive for NF-L was lower in MS patients compared to healthy controls or Sjögren syndrome patients. This finding is in contrast with other studies that describe that antibodies to NF-L are more frequently found in MS patients than in healthy controls (Newcombe *et al.*, 1985, Silber *et al.*, 2002, Ehling *et al.*, 2004). Besides NF-L, only recently a new possible auto-antigen has been discovered in MS patients, contactin-2/TAG-1 (Derfuss *et al.*, 2009). Using a proteomic approach, Derfuss *et al.* identified this axonal protein recognized by both auto-antibodies and T helper (Th) 1 and Th17 cells in MS patients. How these anti-neuronal responses can lead to axonal damage is as yet unclear. However, a role for pathogenic antibodies to neuronal antigens in MS may explain the response of some MS patients to plasma exchange or intravenous Ig (Dau *et al.*, 1980).

EXPERIMENTAL AUTOIMMUNE ENCEPHALOMYELITIS

The first recorded (unintentional) experimentally induced encephalomyelitis was carried out by Louis Pasteur in 1885 while developing a rabies vaccine produced in the brains of live rabbits. Between 1894 and 1914 the vaccine along with the brain components were repeatedly administered in an effort to induce a protective immune response against the rabies virus. While initial studies were considered safe and at least effective in protecting against rabies, later preparations induced varying degrees of paralysis and in the most severe forms mortality in vaccinated subjects. Pathological examination of the CNS revealed extensive inflammation and perivenous demyelination in the brain and spinal cord in some cases. The cause of the paralysis was not due to reaction against the attenuated rabies virus but against the brain antigens in the preparation. It was probably these early human studies and following studies showing induction of paralysis of rabbits could be induced with brain tissues alone (reviewed van Epps, 2005, Baxter, 2007), that stimulated Thomas Rivers studies in rhesus monkeys (Rivers *et al.*, 1933).

In several studies Rivers noted that clinical neurological was associated with inflammation and myelin damage. While Rivers studies required repeated injection of the brain tissues Kabat and colleagues (Kabat *et al.*, 1951) showed that augmenting the immune response using an adjuvant developed by Freund (Freund and Hosmer, 1937) required only a single injection to induce disease - and thus experimental autoimmune encephalomyelitis (EAE) emerged. So immunisation of susceptible animals with CNS antigens gives rise to a spectrum of inflammatory disorders collectively named EAE. Despite the many different clinical courses and pathology due to the sensitization procedure, the auto-antigen of choice and the animal strain used, EAE is the most frequent and intensely used experimental model of MS and has heavily influenced the preclinical development of therapeutic strategies. In particular such approaches have focused on the role of CD4+ helper T cells since several lines of evidence support the held notion that CD4+ T cells play a crucial role in mediating the development of inflammatory lesions in both MS and EAE. This observation has lead to the development of therapeutic interventions that target helper T-cell functions in MS patients and has at least partly positive clinical effects. However, several treatments that were successful in EAE were unsuccessful in MS patients, such as IFN-γ that was found to be protective in EAE (Lublin *et al.*, 1993, Heremans *et al.*, 1996) while it exacerbates disease in humans (Panitch *et al.*, 1987).

Many different models of EAE have been described each having their own specific characteristic, but can be classified as hyperacute, acute, chronic and chronic relapsing. Commonly used animal models are summarized in Table 1. Due to the wide variety of biological tools available, rodent models are the most widely used system to probe the mechanisms underlying MS. Moreover, the extensive numbers of mutant mice deficient in specific immune factors allow detailed investigation of the disease models. The majority of EAE has been induced using myelin- antigens, such as myelin basic protein (MBP), proteolipid protein (PLP), myelin associated glycoprotein (MAG) and MOG. The latter being the most effective although it only represents 2.5 % of the total myelin proteins (Smith *et al.*, 2005).

AUTOIMMUNE MEDIATED NEURONAL DAMAGE

EAE models of MS induced by immunization with myelin proteins or peptides show preferential white matter pathology which is to be expected. However since in MS grey matter pathology is also present and indeed probably contributes to the atrophy and the cognitive problems observed in MS, better animal models reflecting both grey and white matter pathology are more useful to investigate the mechanisms behind this aspect of the disease.

Immunizing animals with neuronal and axonal proteins or peptides induces little more severe axonal pathology, depending on the animal, strain and the antigen. Often the axonal pathology is seen in the spinal cord and can include cellular infiltrates, immunoglobulin and complement deposits.

Table 1. Autoimmune models of multiple sclerosis

Type	Model	Features	References
Autoimmune	Lewis rats: active immunization or T-cell transfer	Monophasic disease, minimal demyelination	Swanborg, 2001
	Dark agouti rats: immunization with MOG or SCH in IFA	Chronic relapsing disease	Lorentzen et al., 1995 Storch et al., 1998
	Biozzi ABH mice: immunization with MOG, PLP, SCH or NF-L	Chronic relapsing disease, acute disease	Amor et al., 2005 Baker et al., 1990 Huizinga et al., 2007
	C57BL/6 mice: immunization with MOG35-55	Chronic progressive disease	Slavin et al., 1998
	Rhesus macaques: immunization with MOG or MBP	Hyperacute disease resembling acute disseminated encephalomyelitis	Kerlero de Rosbo et al., 2000 Van Lambalgen and Jonker, 1987
	Common marmosets: immunized with MOG or human white matter	Progressive or relapsing-remitting disease	Brok et al., 2001 Massacesi et al., 1995
Spontaneous	Humanized transgenic mice with TCR for MBP85-99 and HLA-DR15	High incidence of paralysis after 6 months	Ellmerich et al., 2005
	Transgenic mice with TCR for MOG	Spontaneous optic neuritis	Bettelli et al., 2003

Similar when animals are immunized with myelin antigens, when immunizing animals with neuroaxonal antigens T and B cell responses can be characterized. For example, to examine the pathogenicity of anti-NF-L immune responses, we have demonstrated that immunisation of Biozzi ABH mice with NF-L leads to paralysis and spasticity (Huizinga *et al.*, 2007), debilitating clinical features of MS. In this novel model of axonal damage, which may mimic several features observed in MS, immunoglobulins were observed in the axons in the spinal cord of animals with disease but not in immunised mice that did not exhibit overt clinical signs.

Where immunization with NF-L induced little demyelination, transfer of NF-M 15-35 - specific T cells into native C57BL/6 mice caused, what the authors described as confluent demyelination and severe axonal damage (Krishnamoorthy *et al.,* 2009). They discovered NF-M as a candidate autoantigen by the observation that myelin-specific T cells recognize NF-M in a MOG knock out mice expressing a MOG-specific T cell receptor (TCR). Apparently MOG 35-55 and NF-M 18-30 share essential TCR contact positions. These findings indicate that myelin or neuronal specific T cells could also induce neuronal or myelin damage via cross-reactivity with neuronal or myelin antigens, respectively. This cross-reactivity between reactive T cells and other antigens has been detected before. T lymphocytes recognising synapsin - a highly conserved neuronal protein – were detected in MS patients (Polak *et al.,* 2001). However, in the animal model at least T cells recognising the myelin protein MBP also recognised synapsin (De Santis *et al.,* 1992). Another example of this kind of cross-reactivity is the reactivity of T and B cells to myelin antigens after immunizing Lewis rats with β-synuclein (Mor *et al.,* 2003, Kela-Madar *et al.,* 2009). Furthermore, immunization of C57BL/6 mice with amyloid-β develop an inflammatory disease of the CNS characterized by the presence of perivenular inflammatory foci containing macrophages, T and B cells and immunoglobulin both in the brain and spinal cord (Furlan *et al.,* 2003). Immunization of C57BL/6 mice with a protein involved in Alzheimer's Disease, tau, also caused axonal loss and severe inflammation but interestingly, the authors could not detect demyelination (Rosenmann *et al.,* 2006). Mathey and colleagues investigated the inflammatory response when injecting an antibody directed to neurofascin (NF) in EAE induced DA rats and observed initial axonal pathology and exacerbation of clinical disease, but no enhanced inflammation or demyelination (Mathey *et al.,* 2007). Interestingly, the authors used a monoclonal antibody directed to both NF-155 (myelin-related) and NF-186 (located at Node of Ranvier) isoforms *in vitro*, but could only find binding of the antibody to NF-186 *in vivo*.

Recently, Derfuss and colleagues have shown that T cells reactive to contactin-2/TAG-1, a neuronal protein located at the juxtaparanodal region of myelinated neurons can transfer disease (Derfuss *et al.,* 2009). Preliminary results suggest so far that adoptive transfer of NF-L reactive T cells does not induce disease in Biozzi ABH mice, which may suggest an important role for

Table 2. Axonal pathology in autoimmune animal models

Antigen	Species / type	Clinical disease	Neuropathology	Proposed disease mechanism	References
NF-L	Mouse, Biozzi ABH	Acute disease with spastic paresis and spastic tail	Axonal degeneration, inflammation in dorsal column of spinal cord	Antibody-mediated	Huizinga et al., 2007 Huizinga et al., 2008
NF-M 15-35	Mouse, C57BL/6	Severe EAE	Inflammation in spinal cord, confluent demyelination, severe axonal loss	T-cell mediated	Krishnamoorthy et al., 2009
Contactin-2/ TAG-1	Rat, Dark Agouti	Loss of weight, loss of tail tone, occasional hind limb paralysis	Preferential inflammation of gray matter of the spinal cord and cortex	T-cell mediated	Derfuss et al., 2009
Tau	Mouse, C57BL/6	Limb tail followed by hind leg paresis	Axonal damage, severe inflammation, no demyelination, gliosis	T cell/ antibody-mediated	Rosenmann et al., 2006
β-synuclein 93-111	Rat, Lewis	Paralysis of posterior paws, uveitis	Inflammatory infiltrates in spinal cord	T-cell mediated	Mor et al., 2003

Table 2. (Continued)

Antigen	Species / type	Clinical disease	Neuropathology	Proposed disease mechanism	References
Neurofascin-186	Rat, Dark Agouti	Partial/ complete loss of tail tone, hind limb weakness/ paralysis	Reversible axonal injury, deposition of complement, antibodies at Nodes of Ranvier,	Antibody-mediated	Mathey *et al.*, 2007
Amyloid-β 1-42	Mouse, C57BL/6	Tail paralysis, paresis of hind-limbs	Inflammation in brain and spinal cord, deposits of immunoglobulins, limited demyelination	T- cell mediated	Furlan *et al.*, 2003

NF-L-antibody producing plasma cells (unpublished). Although, direct evidence for this hypothesis is still absent, antibodies have been found to be present inside axons in MS lesions and in neurons in EAE (Slavin *et al.,* 1996, Huizinga *et al.,* 2008). A summary of these models and their pathology can be seen in Table 2.

CONCLUSION

While early studies focussed on the role autoimmunity to myelin in MS and thus the experimental models more recent studies have also identified immune responses to neuronal antigens. Theses later studies show that not only do people with MS develop immune responses to neuronal antigens but that these responses maybe pathogenic. Immunisation of experimental animals with neuronal antigens or passive transfer of neuronal-reactive immunoglobulin from patients selectively induces neuronal degeneration and damage indicting that a similar response may be pathogenic in humans.

The idea that autoimmunity in MS is not restricted to myelin or myelin associated antigens indicates that therapies targeting the autoimmune responses should take into account approaches to inhibit pathogenic responses to neurons.

REFERENCES

Almeras L, Lefranc D, Drobecq H, de Seze J, Dubucquoi S, Vermersch P, Prin L 2004. New antigenic candidates in multiple sclerosis: identification by serological proteome analysis. *Proteomics.* 4: 2184-94.

Amor S, Smith PA, Hart B, Baker D 2005. Biozzi mice: of mice and human neurological diseases. *J. Neuroimmunol.* 65: 1-10.

Amor S, Puentes F, Baker D, van der Valk P 2010. Inflammation in neurodegenerative diseases . *Immunology.* 129: 154-69.

Andersson M, Alvarez-Cermeño J, Bernardi G, Cogato I, Fredman P, Frederiksen J, Fredrikson S, Gallo P, Grimaldi LM, Grønning M, et al 1994. Cerebrospinal fluid in the diagnosis of multiple sclerosis: a consensus report. *J Neurol Neurosurg Psychiatry.* 57: 897-902.

Baker D, O'Neill JK, Gschmeissner SE, Wilcox CE, Butter C, Turk JL 1990. Induction of chronic relapsing experimental allergic encephalomyelitis in Biozzi mice. *J. Neuroimmunol.* 28: 261-70.

Bartos A, Fialová L, Soukupová J, Kukal J, Malbohan I, Pitha J 2007a. Antibodies against light neurofilaments in multiple sclerosis patients. *Acta Neurol. Scand.* 116: 100-7.

Bartos A, Fialová L, Soukupová J, Kukal J, Malbohan I, Pit'ha J 2007b. Elevated intrathecal antibodies against the medium neurofilament subunit in multiple sclerosis. *J. Neurol.* 254: 20-5.

Baxter AG 2007. The origin and application of experimental autoimmune encephalomyelitis. *Nat. Rev. Immunol.* 7: 904-12.

Bettelli E, Pagany M, Weiner HL, Linington C, Sobel RA, Kuchroo VK 2003. Myelin oligodendrocyte glycoprotein-specific T cell receptor transgenic mice develop spontaneous autoimmune optic neuritis. *J. Exp. Med.* 197: 1073-81.

Bergers E, Bot JC, De Groot CJ, Polman CH, Lycklama à Nijeholt GJ, Castelijns JA, van der Valk P, Barkhof F 2002. Axonal damage in the spinal cord of MS patients occurs largely independent of T2 MRI lesions. *Neurology.* 59: 1766-71.

Bitsch A, Schuchardt J, Bunkowski S, Kuhlmann T, Brück W 2000. Acute axonal injury in multiple sclerosis. Correlation with demyelination and inflammation. *Brain.* 123: 1174-83.

Bjartmar C, Kidd G, Mörk S, Rudick R, Trapp BD 2000. Neurological disability correlates with spinal cord axonal loss and reduced N-acetyl aspartate in chronic multiple sclerosis patients. *Ann. Neurol.* 48: 893-901.

Bö L, Dawson TM, Wesselingh S, Mörk S, Choi S, Kong PA, Hanley D, Trapp BD 1994. Induction of nitric oxide synthase in demyelinating regions of multiple sclerosis brains. *Ann. Neurol.* 36: 778-86.

Bö L, Vedeler CA, Nyland H, Trapp BD, Mørk SJ 2003. Intracortical multiple sclerosis lesions are not associated with increased lymphocyte infiltration. *Mult. Scler.* 9: 323-31.

Bö L, Geurts JJ, Mörk SJ, van der Valk P 2006. Grey matter pathology in multiple sclerosis. *Acta Neurol. Scand. Suppl.* 183: 48-50.

Brok HP, Bauer J, Jonker M, Blezer E, Amor S, Bontrop RE, Laman JD, 't Hart BA 2001. Non-human primate models of multiple sclerosis. *Immunol. Rev.* 83: 173-85.

Brorson JR, Schumacker PT, Zhang H 1999. Nitric oxide acutely inhibits neuronal energy production. The Committees on Neurobiology and Cell Physiology. *J. Neurosci.* 19: 147-58.

Brück W, Porada P, Poser S, Rieckmann P, Hanefeld F, Kretzschmar HA, Lassmann H 1995. Monocyte/macrophage differentiation in early multiple sclerosis lesions. *Ann. Neurol.* 38: 788-96.

Charcot JM 1868. Histologie de la sclérose en plaques. *Gaz Hôpital* (Paris). 41: 554-566.

Ciccarelli O, Giugni E, Paolillo A, Mainero C, Gasperini C, Bastianello S, Pozzilli C 1999. Magnetic resonance outcome of new enhancing lesions in patients with relapsing-remitting multiple sclerosis. *Eur. J. Neurol.* 6: 455-9.

Dau PC, Petajan JH, Johnson KP, Panitch HS, Bornstein MB 1980. Plasmapheresis in multiple sclerosis: preliminary findings. *Neurology.* 30: 1023-8.

Derfuss T, Parikh K, Velhin S, Braun M, Mathey E, Krumbholz M, Kümpfel T, Moldenhauer A, Rader C, Sonderegger P, Pöllmann W, Tiefenthaller C, Bauer J, Lassmann H, Wekerle H, Karagogeos D, Hohlfeld R, Linington C, Meinl E 2009. Contactin-2/TAG-1-directed autoimmunity is identified in multiple sclerosis patients and mediates gray matter pathology in animals. *Proc. Natl. Acad. Sci. U. S. A.* 106: 8302-7.

De Santis ML, Roth GA, Cumar FA 1992. Cellular immune crossreactivity between myelin basic protein and synapsin in rats with experimental allergic encephalomyelitis. *J. Neurosci. Res.* 31: 46-51.

DeVries GH 2004. Cryptic axonal antigens and axonal loss in multiple sclerosis. *Neurochem. Res.* 29: 1999-2006.

Ehling R, Lutterotti A, Wanschitz J, Khalil M, Gneiss C, Deisenhammer F, Reindl M, Berger T 2004. Increased frequencies of serum antibodies to neurofilament light in patients with primary chronic progressive multiple sclerosis. *Mult. Scler.* 10: 601-6.

Eikelenboom MJ, Petzold A, Lazeron RH, Silber E, Sharief M, Thompson EJ, Barkhof F, Giovannoni G, Polman CH, Uitdehaag BM 2003. Multiple sclerosis: Neurofilament light chain antibodies are correlated to cerebral atrophy. *Neurology.* 60: 219-23.

Ellmerich S, Mycko M, Takacs K, Waldner H, Wahid FN, Boyton RJ, King RH, Smith PA, Amor S, Herlihy AH, Hewitt RE, Jutton M, Price DA, Hafler DA, Kuchroo VK, Altmann DM 2005. High incidence of spontaneous disease in an HLA-DR15 and TCR transgenic multiple sclerosis model. *J. Immunol.* 174: 1938-46.

Esiri MM, Reading MC 1987. Macrophage populations associated with multiple sclerosis plaques.. *Neuropathology and Applied Neurobiology*, 13: 451–465

Fissolo N, Haag S, de Graaf KL, Drews O, Stevanovic S, Rammensee HG, Weissert R 2009. Naturally presented peptides on major histocompatibility complex I and II molecules eluted from central nervous system of multiple sclerosis patients. *Mol. Cell Proteomics.* 8: 2090-101.

Forooghian F, Cheung RK, Smith WC, O'Connor P, Dosch HM 2007. Enolase and arrestin are novel nonmyelin autoantigens in multiple sclerosis. *J. Clin. Immunol.* 27: 388-96.

Freund J, Hosmer EP 1937. Sensitization and antibody formation after injection of tubercle bacilli and paraffin oil. *Proc. Soc. Exp. Biol. Med.* 37: 509-513

Frischer JM, Bramow S, Dal-Bianco A, Lucchinetti CF, Rauschka H, Schmidbauer M, Laursen H, Sorensen PS, Lassmann H 2009. The relation between inflammation and neurodegeneration in multiple sclerosis brains. *Brain.* 132: 1175-89. .

Frommann C 1878. Untersuchungen über die Gewebsveränderungen bei der Multiplen Sklerose des Gehirns un Rückenmarks. Jena: Verlag von Gustav Fischer. 1-123

Fujinami RS, Oldstone MB 1985. Amino acid homology between the encephalitogenic site of myelin basic protein and virus: mechanism for autoimmunity. *Science.* 230: 1043-5.

Furlan R, Brambilla E, Sanvito F, Roccatagliata L, Olivieri S, Bergami A, Pluchino S, Uccelli A, Comi G, Martino G 2003. Vaccination with amyloid-beta peptide induces autoimmune encephalomyelitis in C57/BL6 mice. *Brain.* 126: 285-91.

Gilmore CP, DeLuca GC, Bö L, Owens T, Lowe J, Esiri MM, Evangelou N 2009. Spinal cord neuronal pathology in multiple sclerosis. *Brain Pathol.* 19: 642-9.

Gimsa U, Peter SV, Lehmann K, Bechmann I, Nitsch R 2000. Axonal damage induced by invading T cells in organotypic central nervous system tissue in vitro: involvement of microglial cells. *Brain Pathol.* 10: 365-77.

Hauser SL, Bhan AK, Gilles F, Kemp M, Kerr C, Weiner HL 1986. Immunohistochemical analysis of the cellular infiltrate in multiple sclerosis lesions. *Ann. Neurol.* 19: 578-87.

Heremans H, Dillen C, Groenen M, Martens E, Billiau A 1996. Chronic relapsing experimental autoimmune encephalomyelitis (CREAE) in mice: enhancement by monoclonal antibodies against interferon-gamma. *Eur. J. Immunol.* 26: 2393-8.

Huizinga R, Heijmans N, Schubert P, Gschmeissner S, 't Hart BA, Herrmann H, Amor S 2007. Immunization with neurofilament light protein induces spastic paresis and axonal degeneration in Biozzi ABH mice. *J. Neuropathol. Exp. Neurol.* 66: 295-304.

Huizinga R, Gerritsen W, Heijmans N, Amor S 2008. Axonal loss and gray matter pathology as a direct result of autoimmunity to neurofilaments. *Neurobiol. Dis.* 32: 461-70. .

Huizinga R, Hintzen RQ, Assink K, van Meurs M, Amor S 2009. T-cell responses to neurofilament light protein are part of the normal immune repertoire. *Int. Immunol.* 21: 433-41.

Höftberger R, Aboul-Enein F, Brueck W, Lucchinetti C, Rodriguez M, Schmidbauer M, Jellinger K, Lassmann H 2004. Expression of major histocompatibility complex class I molecules on the different cell types in multiple sclerosis lesions. *Brain Pathol.* 14: 43-50.

Kabat EA, Wolf A, Bezer AE, Murray JP 1951. Studies on acute disseminated encephalomyelitis produced experimentally in rhesus monkeys. *J. Exp. Med.* 93: 615-33.

Kela-Madar N, de Rosbo NK, Ronen A, Mor F, Ben-Nun A 2009. Autoimmune spread to myelin is associated with experimental autoimmune encephalomyelitis induced by a neuronal protein, beta-synuclein *J. Neuroimmunol.* 208: 19-29.

Kerlero de Rosbo N, Brok HP, Bauer J, Kaye JF, 't Hart BA, Ben-Nun A 2000. Rhesus monkeys are highly susceptible to experimental autoimmune encephalomyelitis induced by myelin oligodendrocyte glycoprotein: characterisation of immunodominant T- and B-cell epitopes. *J. Neuroimmunol.* 110: 83-96.

Kidd D, Barkhof F, McConnell R, Algra PR, Allen IV, Revesz T 1999. Cortical lesions in multiple sclerosis. *Brain.* 122 : 17-26.

Krishnamoorthy G, Saxena A, Mars LT, Domingues HS, Mentele R, Ben-Nun A, Lassmann H, Dornmair K, Kurschus FC, Liblau RS, Wekerle H 2009. Myelin-specific T cells also recognize neuronal autoantigen in a transgenic mouse model of multiple sclerosis. *Nat. Med.* 15: 626-32.

Koch M, Heersema D, Mostert J, Teelken A, De Keyser J 2007. Cerebrospinal fluid oligoclonal bands and progression of disability in multiple sclerosis. *Eur. J. Neurol.* 14: 797-800.

Kolln J, Ren HM, Da RR, Zhang Y, Spillner E, Olek M, Hermanowicz N, Hilgenberg LG, Smith MA, van den Noort S, Qin Y 2006. Triosephosphate isomerase- and glyceraldehyde-3-phosphate dehydrogenase-reactive autoantibodies in the cerebrospinal fluid of patients with multiple sclerosis. *J. Immunol.* 177: 5652-8.

Kutzelnigg A, Lucchinetti CF, Stadelmann C, Brück W, Rauschka H, Bergmann M, Schmidbauer M, Parisi JE, Lassmann H 2005. Cortical demyelination and diffuse white matter injury in multiple sclerosis. *Brain.* 128: 2705-12. .

Lefranc D, Almeras L, Dubucquoi S, de Seze J, Vermersch P, Prin L 2004. Distortion of the self-reactive IgG antibody repertoire in multiple sclerosis as a new diagnostic tool. *J. Immunol.* 172: 669-78.

Lehmann PV, Sercarz EE, Forsthuber T, Dayan CM, Gammon G 1993. Determinant spreading and the dynamics of the autoimmune T-cell repertoire. Immunol. *Today.* 14: 203-8.

Liu JS, Zhao ML, Brosnan CF, Lee SC 2001. Expression of inducible nitric oxide synthase and nitrotyrosine in multiple sclerosis lesions. *Am. J. Pathol.* 158: 2057-66.

Lorentzen JC, Issazadeh S, Storch M, Mustafa MI, Lassman H, Linington C, Klareskog L, Olsson T 1995. Protracted, relapsing and demyelinating experimental autoimmune encephalomyelitis in DA rats immunized with syngeneic spinal cord and incomplete Freund's adjuvant. *J. Neuroimmunol.* 63: 193-205.

Lublin FD, Knobler RL, Kalman B, Goldhaber M, Marini J, Perrault M, D'Imperio C, Joseph J, Alkan SS, Korngold R 1993. Monoclonal anti-gamma interferon antibodies enhance experimental allergic encephalomyelitis. *Autoimmunity.* 16: 267-74.

Massacesi L, Genain CP, Lee-Parritz D, Letvin NL, Canfield D, Hauser SL 1995. Active and passively induced experimental autoimmune encephalomyelitis in common marmosets: a new model for multiple sclerosis. *Ann. Neurol.* 37: 519-30.

Mathey EK, Derfuss T, Storch MK, Williams KR, Hales K, Woolley DR, Al-Hayani A, Davies SN, Rasband MN, Olsson T, Moldenhauer A, Velhin S, Hohlfeld R, Meinl E, Linington C 2007. Neurofascin as a novel target for autoantibody-mediated axonal injury. *J. Exp. Med.* 204: 2363-72.

Medana IM, Gallimore A, Oxenius A, Martinic MM, Wekerle H, Neumann H 2000. MHC class I-restricted killing of neurons by virus-specific CD8+ T lymphocytes is effected through the Fas/FasL, but not the perforin pathway. *Eur. J. Immunol.* 30: 3623-33.

Mews I, Bergmann M, Bunkowski S, Gullotta F, Brück W 1998. Oligodendrocyte and axon pathology in clinically silent multiple sclerosis lesions. *Mult. Scler.* 4: 55-62.

Miller SD, McRae BL, Vanderlugt CL, Nikcevich KM, Pope JG, Pope L, Karpus WJ 1995. Evolution of the T-cell repertoire during the course of experimental immune-mediated demyelinating diseases. *Immunol. Rev.* 144: 225-44.

Mitrovic B, Ignarro LJ, Montestruque S, Smoll A, Merrill JE 1994. Nitric oxide as a potential pathological mechanism in demyelination: its differential effects on primary glial cells in vitro. *Neuroscience.* 61: 575-85.

Mor F, Quintana F, Mimran A, Cohen IR 2003. Autoimmune encephalomyelitis and uveitis induced by T cell immunity to self beta-synuclein. *J. Immunol.* 170: 628-34.

Neumann H, Cavalié A, Jenne DE, Wekerle H 1995. Induction of MHC class I genes in neurons. *Science.* 269: 549-52.

Newcombe J, Gahan S, Cuzner ML 1985. Serum antibodies against central nervous system proteins in human demyelinating disease. *Clin. Exp. Immunol.* 59: 383-90.

Newcombe J, Li H, Cuzner ML 1994. Low density lipoprotein uptake by macrophages in multiple sclerosis plaques: implications for pathogenesis. *Neuropathol. Appl. Neurobiol.* 20: 152-62.

Nitsch R, Pohl EE, Smorodchenko A, Infante-Duarte C, Aktas O, Zipp F 2004. Direct impact of T cells on neurons revealed by two-photon microscopy in living brain tissue. *J. Neurosci.* 24: 2458-64.

Panitch HS, Hirsch RL, Haley AS, Johnson KP 1987. Exacerbations of multiple sclerosis in patients treated with gamma interferon. *Lancet.* 1: 893-5.

Polak T, Schlaf G, Schöll U, Krome-Cesar C, Mäder M, Felgenhauer K, Weber F 2001. Characterization of the human T cell response against the neuronal protein synapsin in patients with multiple sclerosis. *J. Neuroimmunol.* 115: 176-81.

Redwine JM, Buchmeier MJ, Evans CF 2001. In vivo expression of major histocompatibility complex molecules on oligodendrocytes and neurons during viral infection. Am. J. Pathol. 159: 1219-24.

Resnick SM, Pham DL, Kraut MA, Zonderman AB, Davatzikos C 2003. Longitudinal magnetic resonance imaging studies of older adults: a shrinking brain. *J. Neurosci.* 23: 3295-301.

Rindfleisch E 1863. Histologisches Detail zu der grauen Degeneration von Gehirn und Rückenmark. *Arch. Path. Anat. Physiol. Klin. Med.* 26: 474-483

Rivers TM, Sprunt DH, Berry GP 1933. Observations on attempts to produce acute disseminated encephalomyelitis in monkeys. *J. Exp. Med.* 58: 39-53.

Rosenmann H, Grigoriadis N, Karussis D, Boimel M, Touloumi O, Ovadia H, Abramsky O 2006. Tauopathy-like abnormalities and neurologic deficits in mice immunized with neuronal tau protein. *Arch. Neurol.* 63: 1459-67.

Selmaj KW, Raine CS 1988. Tumor necrosis factor mediates myelin and oligodendrocyte damage in vitro. *Ann. Neurol.* 23: 339-46.

Slavin DA, Bucher AE, Degano AL, Soria NW, Roth GA 1996. Time course of biochemical and immunohistological alterations during experimental allergic encephalomyelitis. *Neurochem. Int.* 29: 597-605.

Slavin A, Ewing C, Liu J, Ichikawa M, Slavin J, Bernard CC 1998. Induction of a multiple sclerosis-like disease in mice with an immunodominant epitope of myelin oligodendrocyte glycoprotein. *Autoimmunity.* 28: 109-20.

Smith PA, Heijmans N, Ouwerling B, Breij EC, Evans N, van Noort JM, Plomp AC, Delarasse C, 't Hart B, Pham-Dinh D, Amor S 2005. Native myelin oligodendrocyte glycoprotein promotes severe chronic neurological disease and demyelination in Biozzi ABH mice. *Eur. J. Immunol.* 35: 1311-9.

Storch MK, Stefferl A, Brehm U, Weissert R, Wallström E, Kerschensteiner M, Olsson T, Linington C, Lassmann H 1998. Autoimmunity to myelin oligodendrocyte glycoprotein in rats mimics the spectrum of multiple sclerosis pathology. *Brain Pathol.* 8: 681-94.

Swanborg RH 2001. Experimental autoimmune encephalomyelitis in the rat: lessons in T-cell immunology and autoreactivity. *Immunol. Rev.* 184: 129-35.

Silber E, Semra YK, Gregson NA, Sharief MK 2002. Patients with progressive multiple sclerosis have elevated antibodies to neurofilament subunit. *Neurology.* 58: 1372-81.

Svarcová J, Fialová L, Bartos A, Steinbachová M, Malbohan I 2008. Cerebrospinal fluid antibodies to tubulin are elevated in the patients with multiple sclerosis. *Eur. J. Neurol.* 15: 1173-9.

Terryberry JW, Thor G, Peter JB 1998. Autoantibodies in neurodegenerative diseases: antigen-specific frequencies and intrathecal analysis. *Neurobiol. Aging.* 19: 205-16.

Traugott U, Reinherz EL, Raine CS 1983. Multiple sclerosis. Distribution of T cells, T cell subsets and Ia-positive macrophages in lesions of different ages. *J. Neuroimmunol.* 4: 201-21.

Ulvestad E, Williams K, Vedeler C, Antel J, Nyland H, Mørk S, Matre R 1994. Reactive microglia in multiple sclerosis lesions have an increased expression of receptors for the Fc part of IgG. *J. Neurol. Sci.* 121: 125-31.

Van Epps HL 2005. Thomas Rivers and the EAE model. *J Exp Med.* 202: 4.

Van Lambalgen R, Jonker M 1987. Experimental allergic encephalomyelitis in rhesus monkeys: I. Immunological parameters in EAE resistant and susceptible rhesus monkeys. *Clin. Exp. Immunol.* 68: 100-7.

Werner P, Pitt D, Raine CS 2000. Glutamate excitotoxicity--a mechanism for axonal damage and oligodendrocyte death in Multiple Sclerosis? *J. Neural Transm. Suppl.* 60: 375-85.

Werner P, Pitt D, Raine CS 2001. Multiple sclerosis: altered glutamate homeostasis in lesions correlates with oligodendrocyte and axonal damage. *Ann. Neurol.* 50: 169-80.

Zhang Y, Da RR, Guo W, Ren HM, Hilgenberg LG, Sobel RA, Tourtellotte WW, Smith MA, Olek M, Gupta S, Robertson RT, Nagra R, Van Den Noort S, Qin Y 2005a. Axon reactive B cells clonally expanded in the cerebrospinal fluid of patients with multiple sclerosis. *J. Clin. Immunol.* 25: 254-64.

Zhang Y, Da RR, Hilgenberg LG, Tourtellotte WW, Sobel RA, Smith MA, Olek M, Nagra R, Sudhir G, van den Noort S, Qin Y 2005b. Clonal expansion of IgA-positive plasma cells and axon-reactive antibodies in MS lesions. *J. Neuroimmunol.* 167: 120-30.

Chapter 9

MECHANISMS OF IMMUNE-MEDIATED DAMAGE

Ruth Huizinga[1] and Sandra Amor[2,3]

[1] Department of Immunology, Erasmus MC,
University Medical Center, Rotterdam, The Netherlands.
[2] Department of Pathology, VU Medical Center Amsterdam,
The Netherlands.
[3] Neuroscience and Trauma Centre,
Barts and the London School of Medicine and Dentistry,
Queen Mary University of London, United Kingdom.

ABSTRACT

Understanding the mechanisms driving neuronal degeneration and axonal damage is key to the development of relevant therapies for neurological diseases. In the past several decades a gradual awareness of the different mechanisms involved in neurodegenerative disease such as Alzheimer's' disease, multiple sclerosis, brain trauma, amyotrophic lateral sclerosis and Parkinson's disease has emerged.

Here we first discuss how infections, malignancies and trauma trigger autoimmunity to neurons and axons. Next we review the different mechanisms by which antibodies and T cells induce dysfunction and damage neurons and axons, or conversely, how such pathways could be beneficial in neurodegenerative disorders. Clarification of the different autoimmune mechanisms underlying neurodegeneration will be useful to develop novel therapeutic approaches.

INTRODUCTION

Immune cells, soluble immune molecules such as immunoglobulin, cytokine and chemokines enter the central nervous system (CNS) such as in multiple sclerosis (MS), stroke, infections and trauma or the peripheral nervous system in e.g. Gulllian-Barré syndrome. The assumption that the immune system is pathogenic in these disorders has lead to a number of concepts as to how these responses arise and how the different autoimmune mechanisms operate to induce neuronal and axonal damage.

Autoimmunity in the nervous may arise due to infection with neurotropic viruses such as HIV, HHV6 and JC virus in progressive multifocal leukoencephalopathy as well as other infectious agents. Viral infections have also been suggested to induce autoimmune responses by virtue of mimicking self-antigens, the concept of molecular mimicry, or by stimulating neuronal specific autoreactive T cells present in the periphery.

Disorders which lead to loss of immune tolerance and immune regulation may also lead to development of autoimmunity to neurons and axons, or indeed other CNS antigens in which collateral damage results in neuronal degeneration.

Immune responses to neuronal antigens may arise following the release and presentation of neuronal antigens as a consequence of e.g. trauma, toxins, neurodegeneration, chronic inflammation or infections. The drainage of these antigens to secondary lymph nodes has been suggested to activate, or conversely suppress pre-existing autoreactive cells.

Yet another mechanism involves the phenomenon of 'altered -self' in which the immune system fails to recognise self-proteins either through a lack or loss of immune tolerance or that the self-protein becomes altered and is thus regarded as foreign. In many neurodegenerative disorders mutations in neuronal and axonal proteins give rise to abnormal protein folding and protein aggregation which recognised as foreign triggers an immune response. The presence of these abnormal proteins as well as modified proteins due to oxidative stress for example, is observed in several neurological diseases such as amyotrophic lateral sclerosis (ALS), MS and Alzheimer's disease. In vitro studies and animal models of these disorders reveal that these modified neuronal proteins can activate the innate immune system and, as a consequence may induce autoimmunity. In addition presentation of neuronal antigens in the context of tumours may also trigger immunity to the onco-neuronal antigens. In these so-called paraneoplastic neurological disorders the disease is a direct consequence of immune responses that also recognise structures in the nervous system.

Thus several mechanisms could allow the development of, or induce autoimmunity to neuronal antigens. Here we discuss the various concepts and summarise the major pathways currently suggested to be involved in the development of autoimmunity to neuronal antigens in neurodegenerative disorders. Unravelling these pathways will be crucial to develop relevant therapies aimed to inhibit the pathogenic pathways while aiding the neuroprotective mechanisms.

'INSIDE-OUT' AND 'OUTSIDE-IN' MODELS OF NEURODEGENERATION

Autoimmune-mediated neurodegeneration may arise as a consequence of two pathways. In the so-called 'inside-out' model, autoimmune-mediated damage leads to direct neuronal damage or axonal loss and as a result, the myelin degenerates. In this scenario the pathology should reveal empty myelin sheaths due to an absence of neuronal structures whereas the myelin sheaths are left intact. Alternatively, as observed in the 'outside-in' model, autoimmune responses target the myelin and as a result of direct attack on myelin, naked axons are left vulnerable to damage by, for example, reactive oxygen species (ROS).

INFECTIONS

Virus infections of the CNS can sometimes induce devastating, life-threatening situations as a direct consequence of viral replication in neurons and cell lysis (for review see Amor *et al.,* 2010). Alternatively, viruses may induce programmed cell death of neurons (apoptosis) or a 'dying back' pattern of degeneration or autophagy, due to activation of an intracellular lysosomal-degradation pathway.

Infections of the CNS activate Toll-like receptors (TLR) and Nod-like receptors which initially trigger the innate immune response observed as macrophage and microglia activation. Such responses often involve the release of free radicals by microglia or infiltrating macrophages in an attempt to remove the infectious agent while inducing neuronal damage and neurodegeneration as collateral damage. One consequent of innate immune activation is triggering of the adaptive immune responses that may include autoimmunity to neuronal proteins.

How autoimmunity to neuronal structures develops following neurotropic infections is debatable and controversial. Much of the evidence for the different pathways comes from animal models such as Theiler's murine encephalomyelitis virus (TMEV) and Semliki Forest virus (Table 1) for example. Evidence for cross-reactive immune responses between infectious agents and self-antigens i.e. molecular mimicry has been suggested in both TMEV (Miller *et al.,* 2001) and SFV (Mohktarian *et al.,* 1999) but is nevertheless controversial. Another example of molecular mimicry is that observed in some movement disorders, in which antibodies to group A beta-haemolytic streptococcal infections cross react with human basal ganglia tissue, resulting in motor and psychiatric symptoms (Martino and Giovannoni, 2004). Fortunately the use of antibiotics is very effective.

Table 1. Viruses involved in neurodegenerative disorders

Virus	Pathology	Possible mechanism
Polio	Lower motor neuron loss	Release of neuronal antigens – determinant spreading
Rabies	Neuronal damage	Induces HLA-G expression that may aid immune tolerance and viral latency
HTLV-1	myelopathy/tropical spastic paraparesis	Cross reactivity antibodies with neuronal structures
Herpes virus (HHV6)	Neuronal damage and demyelination	Excessive complement activation, molecular mimicry
EBV	B cell follicles in MS	Antibodies to CNS antigens. Molecular mimicry between viral proteins and CNS antigens
Measles virus	Demyelination	T cells to CNS antigens
LCMV	Inflammation, demyelination	CD8+ T cell killing
TMEV	Demyelination and axonal damage	Presence of antibodies and T cells to myelin antigens
SFV	Demyelination in mice	Antibody and T cell responses to CNS antigens

Viruses may also activate the intrathecal B-cell pool as in Epstein–Barr virus (EBV) infection and this could explain the presence of these antibodies to CNS antigens during infectious mononucleosis (Jilek *et al.,* 2007).

Intriguingly, recent studies suggest that EBV infection in the CNS in MS might be the underlying trigger for the emergence of intrathecal antibodies or due to molecular mimicry with myelin antigens (Lünemann *et al.*, 2008).

'ALTERED-SELF'

Due to number of mechanisms neurons may be regarded as foreign by the immune system with the possibility therefore of inducing an autoimmune attack. Such so-called altered-self antigens arise due to abnormal aggregation, protein misfolding, or due to oxidative and carbonyl stress known to induce modification of proteins and lipids for example glycation of proteins by reducing sugars. Inflammation in the nervous system that by virtue of the high myelin content that is very rich in lipids, can thus induce a cascade of events involving carbonyl and oxidative stress and the modification of lipids as well as proteins, carbohydrates and nucleic acids. Examples of these modifications include advanced glycation end-products (AGE), advanced lipoperoxidation products (ALE) and advanced oxidation protein products (AOPP) (for review see Harris and Amor, 2011).

In Alzheimer's disease (AD) extracellular accumulation of Aβ peptide and abnormally phosphorylated tau protein trigger microglia activation. In animal models and in culture systems such aggregated proteins activate antigen presenting cells. Similar findings are observed in Parkinson's disease (PD) where accumulation of alpha synuclein in neurons leads to profound neurodegeneration. Such accumulation is also observed with dopaminergic neurotoxins such as 6-hydroxydopamine and 1-methyl 4-phenyl 1,2,3,6-tetrahydropyridine (MPTP). In animal models MTPT induces alterations in alpha synuclein leading to accumulations of proteins that trigger CD4 T cells responses although it is unclear if such responses are pathogenic or neuroprotective.

PARANEOPLASTIC DISORDERS

Antineuronal antibodies directed to neuronal antigens expressed by tumour cells frequently lead to neurologic disorders although in many cases disease may occur in the absence of a detectable tumour. As discussed in chapter 4 these cross reactive antibodies are often directed to intracellular antigens. Mechanistically it is difficult to determine how such antibodies gain access to their target inside the neuron. However once inside antibodies may interfere with axonal transport or are involved in protein aggregation or induce dysfunction of the neuron. In some paraneoplastic disorders autoreactive T cells are also observed although it is speculative what roles these autoreactive T cells play in the disease.

TOXINS

Exposure to environmental agents such as neurotoxic agents has also been suggested since autoantibodies to neuronal specific antigens such as neurofilaments have been described in people exposed to lead or mercury and correlated with degree of exposure. In rats such exposure related to the pathology in the nervous system and antibodies purified from humans and rats exposed to this environmental chemical induces neuromuscular dysfunction in experimental animals (El-Fawal et al., 1999).

INDUCTION OF AUTOIMMUNITY

One question is how, following such exposure to infectious agents or environmental neurotoxic agents and neurological damage, does the release of neuronal antigens induce autoimmune responses? Whatever the initial mechanism neuronal proteins and peptides released by damaged cells could well reach the peripheral immune system to augment pre-existing autoreactive cells or trigger de novo responses. How neuronal cells, otherwise present in the immune privileged CNS reach the periphery is not clear and probably depends on the initial insult. Although the CNS lacks lymphatic drainage and this contributes to the so-called 'immune-privilege' status, two major routes of antigen drainage have been suggested.

It is now realised that dendritic cells are able to migrate from the CNS to cervical lymph nodes (CLN) (Hatterer et al., 2006) where they may activate T cells. Alternatively the presence of 'lymphatic structures' in the CNS suggest that antigen presenting cells can come in contact with T cells within the brain itself (Serafini et al., 2006). In MS and EAE, myelin antigens (De Vos et al., 2002) and axonal antigens (van Zwam et al., 2009) are present in the cervical lymph node. These authors also observed that the numbers of cells containing neuronal antigens increases with progression of disease in EAE. Whether the presence of neuronal antigens in the local lymph nodes results in pathogenic autoimmunity or limits an otherwise 'pathogenic responses' is still unclear. Axonal antigens, released in soluble form upon CNS damage (Galea *et al.*, 2007) drain to the regional lymph nodes. Harling-Berg *et al.* (1999) showed that injection of proteins in the ventricles or the brain parenchyma drained to the CLN and this route was very effective for mounting a humoral immune response although the exact pathways require further study.

For pathogenic cells such as T cells, NK cells, macrophages, migration into the CNS relies on a plethora of pathways including upregulation of adhesion molecules and gradients of chemokines and cytokines. Some excellent reviews on cellular entry into the central nervous system are available and not the topic of this review so the reader is directed to Engelhardt (2008) and Carvey *et al.*, (2009).

MECHANISMS OF AUTOIMMUNE MEDIATED NEURONAL INJURY ANTIBODIES, COMPLEMENT AND FC RECEPTORS

Antibodies to self antigens help remove dead cells by enhancing phagocytosis. As a rule antibodies do not reach the CNS due to an intact BBB. In chronic diseases such as MS the scenario is different since the BBB is compromised making it more permeable for antibodies. Similarly during mechanical injury to the brain as in ischemia or brain trauma the BBB is compromised allowing serum antibodies and possible neuron reactive antibodies to reach their target in the CNS.

As discussed in other chapters in this book pathogenic autoimmunity to neuronal structures are present in patients and the question is 'what are the mechanisms by which such responses cause injury to neurons?'

One such way is by interfering with neuronal function. Neurofilaments are synthesised and assembled in neuronal cell bodies, transported along axons and degraded in the synapse. In several pathological diseases such as ALS, diabetic neuropathy and Parkinson's disease, where NF aggregates form Lewy bodies, and in neurofibrillary tangles in Alzheimer's disease, neuronal filaments aggregate in the cell bodies and axons. In peripheral disease such as Charcot-Marie-Tooth syndrome (Brownlees *et al.*, 2002) abnormalities in neurofilament assembly and axonal transport is due to mutations in the protein. Such abnormalities in α-internexin as well as NF have also been identified in neuronal intermediate filament inclusion disease (Momeni *et al.*, 2006). Aggregation of NF proteins may be due to mutations in the proteins themselves, or alternatively immunological mechanisms may induce abnormal function leading to aggregation for example by cross-linking of antibodies recognising neuronal structures. Microinjection of antibodies to kinesin and dynein - proteins involved in axonal transport of NF - in the DRG. in which green fluorescent protein was used to tag NF impaired anterograde and retrograde NF transport (Theiss *et al.*, 2005).

Complement activation may contribute significantly to autoimmune mediated damage in neurodegenerative disorders as a result of antibodies binding to neurons. In the CNS complement components and receptors are expressed by astrocytes, microglia as well as neurons. This is particularly prominent in neurodegenerative disorders where in addition to elimination of aggregated proteins neuronal damage is associated with IgG and complement factor C4 deposition on necrotic cells. For example C1q and C3 are involved in synaptic removal during development and these proteins expressing C3 receptors. That these proteins are increased in the CNS in many neurodegenerative diseases indicates a probable role for complement in neuronal degeneration. This is supported by the finding that aggregated A beta peptides directly activates both the alternative and classical pathway of the complement system in vitro (Rogers *et al.*, 1992) although in humans it is difficult to determine if autoantibodies are involved in such activation. Much of the evidence for complement involvement in neurodegenerative disorders comes from animal models that show both a pathogenic, as well as neuroprotective and neuroregeneration role of complement.

Receptors for Fc (FcR) of immunoglobulin facilitate uptake of immunoglobulin by cells. This mechanism aids the uptake and clearance of, for example, bacteria coated or 'opsonised' with antibodies. Immunoglobulin bound to FcR trigger numerous biological activities in effector cells depending on whether they activate immunoresponsive tyrosine activating motifs (ITAMS) or inhibitory motifs (ITIMs), which are phosphorylated by tyrosine kinases during signal transduction. In the peripheral nervous system FcR are expressed by Schwann cells (Vedeler *et al.*, 1991) and in the CNS FcR are widely expressed by microglia. Few studies have described such expression on neurons in vivo (Andoh and Kuraishi, 2004) although expression of FcR is observed on a neuronal cell line in vitro (Gorini *et al.*, 1992). The high affinity receptor IgG receptor FcgRI is expressed on primary sensory neurons and is activated by Ig-antigen complex which leads to increased intracellular calcium, and release of neurotransmitters. Excessive release is associated with neuronal damage and disease. As described above Ig from ALS patients is taken up by neurons and may enhance neuronal damage by exacerbating neurotransmitter release. Mohamed *et al.* (2002) elegantly showed that F(ab')2 fragments of Ig from ALS patients are not taken up by neurons and thus does not induce neurotransmitter release. Likewise neurons in mice lacking the gamma subunit of the FcR, fail to take up ALS IgG and the acetylcholine release were markedly reduced. Thus targeting this pathway may help in the treatments of ALS but also spasticity and neuronal damage in other neurodegenerative disorders such as MS.

T CELLS AND NEURODEGENERATION

A crucial requirement for CD8+ T cell activation is the presence of Class I major histocompatibility (MHC) antigens while MHC-class II expression is required for activation of CD4+ T cells. Expression of MHC molecules in neurons can be regulated by extrinsic factors as observed following treatment with IFN-gamma where increased expression of MHC-class I on neurons is observed. Conversely electrical activity in neurons limits expression of MHC class I indicating that when electrical transmission is decreased when neurons and axons are damaged, MHC-class I expression is increased rendering these cells more vulnerable to immune attack. The importance of MHC-class I in neuronal death has been described in experimental infections since axonal loss is dramatically reduced while neurological function is improved in MHC-class I knockout mice chronically infected with TMEV (Rivera-Quiñones et al., 1998). As well as viral infections MHC-class I specific T cells activation has also been shown to be involved in EAE where CD8+ T cells are directed to myelin antigens. Also in MS cytotoxic CD8+ T cells are observed in close association with neurons although it is unclear what the cognate antigen is. In inflammation neurons are not merely passive since several studies show that neurons produce IFN-gamma and stimulate apoptosis of T cells (Flügel et al., 2000, Neumann et al., 1997, Olsson et al., 1992). This is possibly reflected by the finding that increased expression of B7.1 and TGF-β1 by neurons is associated with recovery from EAE in mice (Issazadeh et al., 1998).

Conceptually, there are two possible ways that CD8+ T cells damage neurons. Firstly CD8+ T cells directly attack target neurons in a contact-dependent way involving cell: cell interactions. Alternatively they act relatively remotely inducing collateral damage following cytokine secretion. Cell-cell contact involves the secretion of granules containing perforin and serine proteases. Perforins are inserted into the plasma membrane of the neuron forming pores allowing the serine proteases to enter. Once inside the neuron the serine proteases cleave caspases and initiates apoptosis.

Alternatively cytotoxic cells that express CD95 (Fas) mediate CD95–CD95L (Fas ligand) interaction. Neurons express CD95 and after recognizing neuronal antigen-specifically via MHC class I, CD95L signaling activates apoptosis of the neuron. Finally the secretion of the TNF family of cytokines allows binding of TNFα to its receptor TNFR1. Such binding activates the receptor's death domain and initiates apoptosis pathway.

CD8+ T cells produce IL-17, (Tc17 cells) and these augment tissue damage indicating that if cells are present in neurodegenerative disorders they could augment neuronal damage. Compared to CD8 T cells that produce IFN gamma (so called Tc1 cells) known to regulate disease in EAE suggests that such neuronal specific response could also be protective. More recent studies do indeed indicate the role of CD8+ T cell in suppression of neuroantigen specific CD4+ T cells. In MS increased levels of CD8+T cells correlate with disease recovery post-relapse while levels are significantly decreased during episodes of neurological deficit (Baughman et al., 2011). In Rasmussen's syndrome CD8+ T cells are found alongside neurons expressing MHC I and cytotoxic granules in T cells are directed to neurons in the absence of FasL expression (Schwab, 2009). As well as the role of antibodies in PNND cytotoxic T cells recognize the onco-neuroal antigen cdr2. As described in chapter 4 also in ALS, and AD significant numbers of CD8 positive T cells are observed in the close vicinity of neurons although further studies are required to clarify whether these cells are indeed pathogenic.

As well as direct killing by CD8+ T cells, CD4 T cells may also be involved in axonal and neuronal damage by for example aiding production of pathogenic antibodies. In addition T cells may activate macrophages and microglia thus aiding production of reactive oxygen species and mitochondrial dysfunction in neurons.

In summary several pathways have been described for autoimmune mediated damage of neurons. While neuronal antigens could be made available to the immune responses following e.g. viral infection or ischemia, there is little evidence that such antigens draining to the local lymph nodes induce a further rounds of immune activation. Rather such responses are probably protective. Clearly some T cells and antibodies are pathogenic and further studies are available to determine how common these responses are in neurodegenerative diseases in general.

REFERENCES

Amor S, Puentes F, Andoh T and Kuraishi Y 2004. Expression of Fc epsilon receptor I on primary sensory neurons in mice. *Neuroreport.* 15: 2029-31.

Baker D, van der Valk P. Inflammation in neurodegenerative diseases. *Immunology.* 2010 129:154-69.

Baughman EJ, Mendoza JP, Ortega SB, Ayers CL, Greenberg BM, Frohman EM, Karandikar NJ 2011. Neuroantigen-specific CD8+ regulatory T-cell function is deficient during acute exacerbation of multiple sclerosis. *J. Autoimmun.*

Brownlees J, Ackerley S, Grierson AJ, Jacobsen NJ, Shea K, Anderton BH, Leigh PN, Shaw CE and Miller CC 2002. Charcot-Marie-Tooth disease neurofilament mutations disrupt neurofilament assembly and axonal transport. *Hum. Mol. Genet.* 11: 2837-44.

Carvey PM, Hendey B, Monahan AJ.The blood *J. Neurochem.* 2009 111: 291-314.

De Vos AF, van Meurs M, Brok HP, Boven LA, Hintzen RQ, van der Valk P, Ravid R, Rensing S, Boon L, t Hart BA and Laman JD 2002. Transfer of central nervous system autoantigens and presentation in secondary lymphoid organs. *J. Immunol.* 169: 5415-23.

El-Fawal HA, Waterman SJ, De Feo A and Shamy MY 1999. Neuroimmunotoxicology: humoral assessment of neurotoxicity and autoimmune mechanisms. *Environ. Health Perspect.* 107 Suppl 5: 767-75.

Engelhardt B 2008. Immune cell entry into the central nervous system *J. Neurol. Sci.* 274: 23-6.

Flügel A, Schwaiger FW, Neumann H, Medana I, Willem M, Wekerle H, Kreutzberg GW, Graeber MB 2000. Neuronal FasL induces cell death *Brain Pathol.* 10: 353-64.

Fontana A, Gast H, Reith W, Recher M, Birchler T, Bassetti CL 2010. Narcolepsy: autoimmunity, effector T cell activation due to infection, or T cell independent, major histocompatibility complex class II induced neuronal loss? *Brain.* 133(Pt 5):1300-11.

Fotheringham J, Jacobson S 2005. Human herpesvirus 6 and multiple sclerosis: potential mechanisms for virus-induced disease. *Herpes.* 12: 4-9.

Galea I, Bechmann I and Perry VH 2007. What is immune privilege (not)? *Trends Immunol.* 28: 12-8.

Gorini G, Ciotti MT, Starace G, Vigneti E and Raschella G 1992. Fc gamma receptors are expressed on human neuroblastoma cell lines: lack of correlation with N-myc oncogene activity. *Int. J. Neurosci.* 62: 287-97.

Harling-Berg CJ, Park TJ and Knopf PM 1999. Role of the cervical lymphatics in the Th2-type hierarchy of CNS immune regulation. *J. Neuroimmunol.* 101: 111-27.

Harris RA, Amor S 2010. Sweet and Sour - Oxidative and Carbonyl Stress in Neurological Disorders. *CNS Neurol Disord Drug Targets.*

Hatterer E, Davoust N, Didier-Bazes M, Vuaillat C, Malcus C, Belin MF and Nataf S 2006. How to drain without lymphatics? Dendritic cells migrate from the cerebrospinal fluid to the B-cell follicles of cervical lymph nodes. *Blood.* 107: 806-12.

Heijmans N, Smith PA, Morris-Downes MM, Pryce G, Baker D, Donaldson AV, t Hart B and Amor S 2005. Encephalitogenic and tolerogenic potential of altered peptide ligands of MOG and PLP in Biozzi ABH mice. *J. Neuroimmunol.* 167: 23-33.

Issazadeh S, Navikas V, Schaub M, Sayegh M, Khoury S 1998. Kinetics of expression of costimulatory molecules *J. Immunol.* 161: 1104-12.

Jilek S, Kuhle J, Meylan P, Reichhart MD, Pantaleo G, Du Pasquier RA 2007. Severe post-EBV encephalopathy *J. Neuroimmunol.* 192: 192-7. 5

Kierdorf K, Wang Y, Neumann H 2010. Immune-mediated CNS damage.Results Probl Cell Differ.51: 173-96

Lünemann JD, Jelcić I, Roberts S, Lutterotti A, Tackenberg B, Martin R, Münz C 2008. EBNA1-specific T cell *J. Exp. Med.* 205: 1763-73.

Martino D, Giovannoni G 2004. Antibasal ganglia antibodies and their relevance to movement disorders. *Curr. Opin. Neurol.* 17: 425-32.

Miller SD, Katz-Levy Y, Neville KL, Vanderlugt CL 2001. Virus-induced autoimmunity *Adv. Virus Res.*56: 199-217..

Mokhtarian F, Zhang Z, Shi Y, Gonzales E, Sobel RA 1999. Molecular mimicry between a viral peptide and a myelin oligodendrocyte glycoprotein peptide induces autoimmune demyelinating disease in mice. *J. Neuroimmunol.* 95(1-2): 43-54.

Mohamed HA, Mosier DR, Zou LL, Siklos L, Alexianu ME, Engelhardt JI, Beers DR, Le WD and Appel SH 2002. Immunoglobulin Fc gamma receptor promotes immunoglobulin uptake, immunoglobulin-mediated calcium increase, and neurotransmitter release in motor neurons. *J. Neurosci. Res.* 69: 110-6.

Momeni P, Cairns NJ, Perry RH, Bigio EH, Gearing M, Singleton AB and Hardy J 2006. Mutation analysis of patients with neuronal intermediate filament inclusion disease (NIFID). *Neurobiol. Aging.* 27: 778 e1-778 e6.

Neumann H, Schmidt H, Wilharm E, Behrens L, Wekerle H 1997. Interferon gamma gene expression *J. Exp. Med.* 186: 2023-31.

Olsson T 1992. Cytokines in neuroinflammatory disease: role of myelin *J. Neuroimmunol.* 40: 211-8.

Pryce G, O'Neill JK, Croxford JL, Amor S, Hankey DJ, East E, Giovannoni G and Baker D 2005. Autoimmune tolerance eliminates relapses but fails to halt progression in a model of multiple sclerosis. *J. Neuroimmunol.* 165: 41-52.

Rivera-Quiñones C, McGavern D, Schmelzer JD, Hunter SF, Low PA, Rodriguez M 1998. Absence of neurological deficits following extensive demyelination *Nat. Med.* 4:187-93.

Rogers J, Cooper NR, Webster S, Schultz J, McGeer PL, Styren SD, Civin WH, Brachova L, Bradt B, Ward P 1992. Complement activation by beta-amyloid in Alzheimer disease. *Proc. Natl. Acad. Sci. U. S. A.* 89: 10016-20.

Schwab N, Bien CG, Waschbisch A, Becker A, Vince GH, Dornmair K, Wiendl H 2009. CD8+ *Brain.* 5: 1236-46.

Serafini B, Rosicarelli B, Magliozzi R, Stigliano E, Capello E, Mancardi GL and Aloisi F 2006. Dendritic cells in multiple sclerosis lesions: maturation stage, myelin uptake, and interaction with proliferating T cells. *J. Neuropathol. Exp. Neurol.* 65: 124-41.

Theiss C, Napirei M and Meller K 2005. Impairment of anterograde and retrograde neurofilament transport after anti-kinesin and anti-dynein antibody microinjection in chicken dorsal root ganglia. *Eur. J. Cell Biol.* 84: 29-43.

van Zwam M, Huizinga R, Melief MJ, Wierenga-Wolf AF, van Meurs M, Voerman JS, Biber KP, Boddeke HW, Hopken UE, Meisel C, Meisel A, Bechmann I, Hintzen RQ, t Hart BA, Amor S, Laman JD and Boven LA 2009. Brain antigens in functionally distinct antigen-presenting cell populations in cervical lymph nodes in MS and EAE. *J. Mol. Med.* 87: 273-86.

Vedeler CA, Matre R, Kristoffersen EK and Ulvestad E 1991. IgG Fc receptor heterogeneity in human peripheral nerves. *Acta Neurol .Scand.* 84: 177-80.

Chapter 10

PERSPECTIVES FOR THERAPY IN NEURODEGENERATIVE DISORDERS

Ruth Huizinga[1] and Sandra Amor[2,3]
[1] Department of Immunology, Erasmus MC,
University Medical Center, Rotterdam, The Netherlands.
[2] Department of Pathology, VU Medical Center Amsterdam,
The Netherlands.
[3] Neuroscience and Trauma Centre,
Barts and the London School of Medicine and Dentistry,
Queen Mary University of London, United Kingdom.

ABSTRACT

New insights into the mechanisms underlying immune-mediated neurodegenerative disorders indicate that therapeutic strategies should not only target the pathogenic immune response but also aid neuroprotection and neuronal repair. In this chapter we review the therapies that are currently used for neurodegenerative disorders including amyotrophic lateral sclerosis, Alzheimer's disease, brain trauma, multiple sclerosis, paraneoplastic neurodegenerative disorders and Parkinson's disease. We first focus on those approaches that target the immune response in disorders in which the immune responses has been shown to play a key role in the disease such as myasthenia gravis, paraneoplastic disorders and multiple sclerosis. In the second part the neuroprotective approaches are discussed including existing approved compounds as well as experimental approaches to treat these disorders.

INTRODUCTION

The mechanisms underlying the progressive neurodegeneration observed in disorders such as Alzheimer's' disease (AD), multiple sclerosis (MS), brain trauma, amyotrophic lateral sclerosis (ALS) and Parkinson's disease (PD) have gained increasing attention not least because of the increase in the aging community. With many more people living into the 9th decade of life and beyond the burden of neurodegenerative disorders is becoming increasingly obvious. In the previous chapters we have outlined the role of the innate and the adaptive immunity in these disorders (see also Amor *et al.,* 2010, Harris and Amor, 2010). The awareness and understanding of pathogenic mechanisms operating in inflammatory and neurodegenerative disorders is key to the development of effective therapies. In many human neurodegenerative disorders the role of the immune response has been extrapolated from animal models of disease. In some cases these models have been crucial for the development of therapies in humans while for others the models are either unavailable or that therapies in the animal models do not translate to the human condition. For example in MS many approaches have proved highly effective in inhibiting clinical and pathological signs of EAE in mice, rats and non-human primates but have proved of little value in the human disease (Amor *et al.,* 2005, Baker and Amor, 2010, Vesterinen *et al.,* 2010).

The idea that many neurodegenerative disorders involve common pathways has allowed direct translation of effective therapies in one disorder to other conditions. Here we review approaches used to inhibit neurodegeneration and aid neuroprotection including the approved compounds and experimental studies in animals. The major groups of therapies are discussed and in each we specifically review the efficacy in different neurodegenerative disorders where known.

THERAPEUTIC APPROACHES

In immune-mediated disorders of the CNS the first line approach is clearly to target the immune response. These therapies are usually non-specific and involve injections to limit or modulate the global immune responses. Understandably this approach may give rise to side effects such as infections due to the non-specificity of broad immunosuppression. Secondly, where the pathogenic component of the immune response is known the therapy can be more specific. For example the use of intravenous immunoglobulin (IVIg) is used to block pathogenic antibodies in paraneoplastic disorders. In MS, widely considered to be an autoimmune T-cell mediated disease, tolerance strategies targeting the pathogenic T cells have been attempted in an effort to ablate the pathogenic T cell and encourage protective and regulatory T cells. Finally therapies that aid protection or repair or replace damaged neurons are crucial particularly in established disease. Clearly such neuroprotective and repair approaches should be used in combination with immunosuppressive therapies.

IMMUNOSUPPRESSIVE THERAPIES

Broad spectrum immunosuppressive first line therapies are usually administered by injection although several have now been developed for oral administration. In MS such therapies include cladribine and teriflunomide, two antiproliferative agents that operate by interfering with metabolic or signalling pathways in activated immune cells. Cladribine, the first orally approved drug for MS is a synthetic chlorinated deoxyadenosine analogue biologically active in selected cells (Leist and Weissert, 2011). It reduces circulating T and B lymphocytes due to accumulation of cladribine phosphates where there is high ratio of deoxycytidine kinase to 5'-nucleotidases. This compound incorporates into DNA interfering with DNA synthesis and repair. The drug also inhibits DNA polymerase and ribonucleotide reductase leading to DNA strand breaks and cell death. Similarly mitoxantrone, a chemotherapeutic agent is also used in MS in which it ablates lymphocytes thought to be instrumental in the pathology. In myasthenia gravis (MG) corticosteroids such as azathioprine remains to be the first line of defense although other drugs such as mycophenolate mofetil have been reported to be more efficacious.

Immunosuppressive therapies have also been attempted in disorders not classically considered to be immune-mediated. For example in ALS several lines of immunosuppressive therapy have been attempted (Calvo et al., 2010). Although general immunosuppressive therapy with cyclophosphamide or total lymphocyte depletion has been used in ALS there is no or limited benefit to patients (Brown et al., 1986, Drachman et al., 1994). Similarly immune-suppressive therapies have been used in PD although here their mode of operation is thought to be via the generation of neuroprotective factors (Lu et al., 2010). Interferon-β (IFNβ) is also a fist line drug for MS in which the mechanism of action has been proposed include immunosuppression and thus beneficial in early MS. As such there is little effect directly on the neurodegenerative component in MS.

Selective Immunosuppression

With the anticipated side effects such as the increased susceptibility to infections following broad spectrum immunosuppression more selective therapies would be advantageous. Such approaches include targeting specific pathways involved the migration of cells into the CNS or blocking the specific pathogenic antibody or T cells thought to be involved in the disease.

In MS approaches inhibiting the migration of cells into the CNS is clearly demonstrable with the use of Tysabri (Nataluzimab) (Comi, 2009) a monoclonal antibody directed to VLA4 that thus blocks entry of all cells expressing this adhesion molecule whether they may be involved in MS or not. More recently Gunnarsson and colleagues (Gunnarsson et al., 2011) indicate that Nataluzimab reduces axonal damage although whether this is secondary to inhibition of the inflammatory responses is unclear. While slightly more specific than broad spectrum immunosuppression, immunity is still necessary to inhibit CNS infections indicting that targeting the immune response is a delicate balance between inhibiting neurodegeneration while allowing sufficient protection against infectious agents and tumours. This may explain why a small number of patients using Tysabri develop the fatal disease progressive multifocal leukoencephalopathy (PML) due to JC virus (Clifford et al., 2010). Similarly inhibiting activated cells, including the supposed pathogenic T cells leaving the lymph nodes and thus not being able to enter the CNS is one mode of action of Gilenya (FTY720 /Fingolimod) (Brinkmann et al., 2010). Both approaches are effective in part in that the symptoms of the disease are significantly diminished. Other mechanisms used to reduce T cells include the monoclonal antibody alemtuzumab. This mAb directed to CD52 expressed on the surface of mature lymphocytes, monocytes, macrophage and some dendritic cells is beneficial in early MS (Minagar et al., 2010) but so far has little effect in the neurodegeneration. That alemtuzumab has been linked to side effects has promoted the use of daclizumab, a mAb to CD25, the a-subunit of the interleukin-2-receptor (IL-2R) on T cells. However rather than depleting T cells it is thought to act by enhancing regulatory NK cells (Bielekova and Becker, 2010).

Yet more specific therapies specifically targeting T cells to myelin protein and myelin peptides have been very effective in inhibit early disease in autoimmune models of MS such approaches are less effective in established disease and in MS itself. Application of such 'tolerance' approaches using oral or intranasal route of administration of antigens have been attempted with the aim of switching the pathogenic responses to a protective one. Such therapies are successful when used in the early stages of EAE in animals but not in the secondary progressive stage (Heijmans *et al.*, 2005, Pryce *et al.*, 2005, Smith *et al.*, 2005). Whether these strategies are effective in MS is under investigation.

The use of altered peptide ligands, again with the same idea of immune deviation has been used in MS. One such approach is glatiramer acetate (Copaxone, copolymer 1), a prescribed therapy for multiple sclerosis. Here it is thought that random peptides mimicking myelin protein modify or deviate the pathogenic response aiding regulatory T cells thereby inhibiting disease in MS (Racke *et al.*, 2010). Such therapies that encourage anti-inflammatory cytokines such as IL-10 and TGF beta, as well as T regs are partially effective in models of PD protecting against neuronal loss. Copaxone has been used in animal models of both ALS and PD (Angelov *et al.*, 2003, Benner *et al.*, 2004).

In short, while variable, little effect has been observed with such antigen specific approaches in MS either because the pathogenic response is not directed to myelin proteins or that the immune response maybe difficult to control. Since antibodies to neuronal and axonal antigens or indeed heat shock proteins may have a pathogenic role in neurological diseases, tolerance strategies should also target other CNS antigens other than myelin in MS.

Antibodies and B cells

For several disorders such as MG and paraneoplastic disorders, removing the source of antibody (tumour) or blocking antibodies has proved highly effective (for review see Pelosof *et al.*, 2010, Farrugia and Vincent, 2010). One approached mentioned above is the use of IVIg proved to be effected in MG, GBS, Stiff person syndrome, Miller-Fisher syndrome, Limbic encephalitis, LEMS, as well as MS (Gold and Kieseier, 2006). IVIg also has a beneficial albeit slight effect, in diabetic patients presenting with axonal damage and while effective in MS although it is unclear whether IVIg impacts on the axonal damage.

More specifically where the specific pathogenic antibody has been identified (or thought to be important) as in MS for example studies have indicated that recombinant antibody fragments maybe useful as autoantibody antagonists to treat the disease (Amor and 't Hart, 2003).

Similarly targeting B cells using Rituximab, a chimaeric IgG k monoclonal antibody to CD20 depletes B cells offer great promise in a number of neurological disorders including MG and MS. In some conditions Rituximab has been shown to reduce number of plasma cells (Huang *et al.,* 2010) although the major effect is depleting CD20 B cells. In MS such depletion does not impact on the oligoclonal bands of Ig and thus pathogenic antibodies. Here the effect is thought to be reduction of the number of B cells which act as antigen presenting cells thereby limiting T cell activation.

Complement and Complement Fixing Antibodies

In contrast to inhibiting pathogenic antibodies several studies indicate that augmenting the immune system to clear protein aggregates is emerging as a promising approach to treat neurodegenerative diseases. For example in AD clinical trials have used both active and passive immunotherapy directed to amyloid-β (Aβ) peptide but this has very little effect on tau accumulations (Citron, 2010). However using a novel animal model Boutajangout and colleagues show that immunotherapy targeting pathological tau is also effective in tauopathies suggesting that this novel approach can also be applied in humans (Boutajangout *et al.,* 2010).

In MG the pathogenic antibodies have been shown to be complement fixing and thus targeting the complement pathway using recombinant C5 complement inhibitor has been shown to be effective in animal models of MG.

Targeting the Innate Immune Response

Microglia activation observed in many neurodegenerative disorders leads to NO and superoxide production as well as IL-1 beta and TNF alpha. NO and superoxide production induces neuronal damage *in vitro* and thus approaches to block these pathways by enhanced anti-oxidants pathways are obvious. Antioxidants such as flavonoids found in green tea (EGCG) protects neurons from apoptosis and reduces neurological damage observed in EAE. Dietary flavonoids and polyphenols found in fruits, vegetables, and spices such as curcumin have been shown to impart neuroprotection in experimental systems and have been suggested to aid protection from dementias (Craggs and Kalaria, 2010). Other approaches include the use of polyunsaturated fatty acids suggested to have a protective effective in models of MS (Harbige *et al.,* 1995, 1997) by augmenting protective cytokines (Harbige *et al.,* 2000).

Targeting the innate immune responses thought to be instrumental in induction of MS lesions (van der Valk and Amor, 2009, van Noort *et al.*, 2010) could also be achieved by examining the natural neuroprotective phenomenon observed in so-called preactive MS lesions. In these early lesions oligodendrocyte stress and resistant to oxidative stress induced apoptosis is suggested by the expression of the heat shock protein alpha B crystallin (van Noort *et al.*, 2010). These studies have shown that *in vitro* this small heat shock proteins induces microglia to adopt a protective phenotype indicating that this might also occur *in vivo*.

NEUROREGENERATION

Restoring Myelin Support

As discussed in chapter 8 and chapter 9 neurodegeneration may arise due to loss of trophic support of myelin. Myelin is essential for the very rapid neuronal transmission. The lack of myelin or limited remyelination that is seen in MS leads to high energy demands by the neuron often leading to degeneration. The limited remyelination may arise due to the loss of oligodendrocyte progenitor cells or due the presence of factors that negatively regulate myelination. Thus one approach to aid myelination is stem cell therapies aimed to increase the numbers of oligodendrocyte progenitor cells. The use of insulin-like growth factor that promotes growth and maturation of oligodendrocytes has also been shown to aid remyelination (Kumar *et al.*, 2007). Interestingly, Gilenya (see above) is also thought to act within the CNS thus having a secondary effect in MS additional to inhibition of lymphocyte trafficking (Brinkmann *et al.*, 2010).

Another approach to aid neuroregeneration is to block the myelin inhibition pathways that operate to prevent aberrant neuronal sprouting. These include Nogo-A, myelin associated glycoprotein and oligodendrocyte myelin glycoprotein. A receptor for Nogo-A is the protein - leucine rich repeat and Ig domain containing-1 - LINGO-1 expressed on neurons during neuronal cone formation. Evidence from animal models of MS suggests that either blocking these inhibitory pathways aids neuronal growth that this maybe useful in MS and spinal cord injury (Simonen *et al.*, 2003; Fontoura *et al.*, 2004). For example LINGO-1 antagonists lead to functional recovery without impacting on the immune system.

That the receptor of Nogo-A (Ng-R) signals through Rho GTPase, the intracellular messenger that mediates the effects of axonal growth, has prompted the development of inhibitors compounds that inactivate the Rho pathway to promote neurite outgrowth. One of these Cethrin a recombinant protein based on bacterial toxin has good neuroprotective and neuroregenerative effects in preclinical studies indicting promise in humans (Baptiste *et al.,* 2009). These approaches thus need to balance augmentation of neuroregeneration with remyelination strategies and as such maybe difficult to balance in human disorders.

Neuronal Growth Factors and Stem Cells

Similar to replacement of OPC, several studies indicate that neuronal networks can be reinstated following augmentation of neural stems cells. For example, while still experimental the use of erythropoietin (Epo) usually used to treat anaemia has been examined in experimental models. Epo and the receptor for Epo is widely expressed in the CNS and is beneficial in neurological disease in ischemia, trauma and epilepsy (Chang *et al.,* 2008). Neuropoietic cytokines such as leukaemia-inhibitory factor (LIF) and ciliary neurotropic factor (CNTF) have also shown promise in axonal injury models enhancing neuronal survival (Blesch *et al.,* 1999).

Alternatively, approaches to augment the neural cells stem differentiation by regulating epigenetic signals such as Sirt1 (silent information regulator 1) a member of the NAD(+) -dependent protein deacetylases. The interest in such epigenetic factors has stimulated development of small-molecule activators of Sirt-1 such as resveratrol and SRT1720 (Dittenhafer-Reed *et al.,* 2011). It remains to be determined if these approaches can be made sufficiently specific to aid neurodegeneration.

In MS and EAE several lines of evidence indicate that proinflammatory mediators such as IFN gamma inhibit neural stem cell differentiation by inhibiting sonic hedgehog pathway. This may not only be restricted to MS but may also be applicable to several neurodegenerative disorders in which persistent inflammation is observed.

Neuroprotective Therapies

Increased expression of sodium, potassium and calcium channels all lead to influx of ions into the axons with the possibility to lead to axonal damage and neurodegeneration and thus blockers of these channels have the potential to inhibit neurodegeneration. As a result of demyelination sodium channels are increased to aid conduction yet persistent expression leads to increased energy demands. Inhibition of sodium channels by blockers such as phenytoin, an anticonvulsant has shown therapeutic efficacy in EAE. In addition phenytoin also interferes with inflammation reducing the function of activated Na+ v1.5 channel on microglia. Other sodium channel blockers are lamotrigine, for use in SP-MS and the anti-arrhythmic agent flecainide. Potassium channel blockers are also effective in restoring impulse conduction in injured axons. Thus targets have also included the potassium TWIK-related acid-sensitive potassium channels which allow the regulated efflux of potassium ions reducing signs of EAE in animals (Bittner et al., 2009, Shi and Sun, 2011). Attenuation of calcium channels have been used with some success in EAE including bepridil, a broad spectrum calcium channel blocker and nitrendipine, a blocker of L-type voltage-gated calcium channels. Nimodipine, nifedipine and ryanodine that block the downstream release of calcium have also been shown to be neuroprotective as has the calpain inhibitor CYLA.

Acid-sensing ion channel (ASIC1) contributes to axonal dysfunction and degeneration in inflammatory lesions by augmenting neuronal Na+ and Ca2+ influxes during tissue acidosis, and experimental ASIC1 blockade by the compound amiloride has been shown to inhibit axonal damage in EAE.

Anti-Excitotoxic Agents (Glutamate Blockers)

Glutamate is the main excitatory CNS neurotransmitter, and neuronal toxicity due to excess glutamate is implicated in neurodegenerative disorders. The two glutamate receptors in the CNS are ionotropic named by the agnostic molecule to which they are directed i.e. NMDA, AMPA (aamino-3-hydroxyl-5-methyl-4-isoxazole-propionate) or kainite and the metabotropic receptors. Demyelinated axons also acquire AMPA receptors that in excess allow accumulation of intracellular sodium and calcium. Thus several therapeutic approaches have been developed that block the ionotropic receptor NMDA (N-methyl-D-aspartic acid), AMPA receptor and metabotropic receptor and kainite blockers. For example memantine, a NMDA antagonist is used in AD and is effective in EAE while riluzole used in ALS, inhibits the release of glutamate and modulates kainite and NMDA receptors. In addition flupirirtine, protects neurons against excitotoxic or ischemic damage (Rupalla *et al.*, 1995) and reduce neuronal damage in optic neuritis and ischemia as well as TRAIL induced neuronal damage (Block *et al.*, 1997, Sattler *et al.*, 2008).

Table 1. Immunosuppressive Therapies for Neurodegenerative Disorders

Compound	Mode of action*	Disease
Interferon beta (IFN-β 1a and 1b)	Immunomodulation of pathogenic T cells, decreases MHC class II and MMP9 expression	CIS, RRMS, SPMS
Glatiramer acetate (GA, Copolymer-1)	Immunomodulation enhances Th2 responses, promotes anti-inflammatory response.	CIS, RRMS, Models of ALS and PD
Compound	Mode of action*	Disease
Nataluzimab (Tysabri)	Inhibiting migration of T cells into the CNS.	RRMS, SPMS
Rituximab	B cell depletion but does not deplete plasma cells. Thought to inhibit antigen presenting capacity of B cells thereby inhibiting T cell activation.	MS, MG
Gilenya (Fingolimod; FTY720)	Inhibiting pathogenic cells leaving lymph nodes and suggested to promote remyelination.	MS
Daclizumab	Antibody to CD25 (alpha subunit of IL-2R)	MS
Alemtuzimab	Humanised antibody to CD52. Depletes T and B cells, increased T regs and CD56 NK cells.	MS
Cladribine	anti proliferative by disrupting DNA synthesis and repair.	MS
Teriflunomide	anti proliferative	MS
Mitoxantrone	Immunosuppressive	MS
Intravenous immunoglobulin (IVIg)	Competition for pathogenic antibodies	MS, MG, GBS, Miller-Fisher syndrome
Laquinimod	Immunomodulatory. Encouragers shift fromproinflammatory Th1 to anti-inflammatory Th2	MS
Non-steroid anti-inflammatories		Parkinson's disease,

* See text for full explanation and references
CIS – clinically isolated syndrome
GBS – Guillian-Barré syndrome.

Another approach to develop antagonists of glutamate receptors involves the kynurenine pathway suggested to be involved in several neurodegenerative disorders including Huntington's (Thevandavakkam *et al.,* 2010); MS (Rajda *et al.,* 2007), ALS (Chen *et al.,* 2009, 2010) and AD (Kincses *et al.,* 2010). The kynurenine pathway involves three compounds that are neuroactive metabolites, the neurotoxins 3-hydroxykynurenine and quinolinic acid, and the neuroprotectant kynurenic acid. Thus targeting this pathway has revealed several compounds that may aid neuroprotection in these disorders (Stone, 2000).

Cannabinoids

The role of cannabinoids in neurodegenerative disorders has been suggested to be immune suppressive and neuroprotective operating by modulating glutamate as well as antioxidative effects (Ortega-Gutiérrez *et al.,* 2005). Exogenous agonists of the cannabinoid CB1-receptor are neuroprotective in EAE (Pryce *et al.,* 2003) and may also be effective in ALS (Rossi *et al.,* 2010).

In conclusion approaches to inhibit inflammation must consider not only the detrimental effects of immunity but also the protective and regenerative effects of the immune response. The increasing knowledge of the role of both the innate immune response such and regulatory T cells in neuroprotection will inevitably expand the numbers of therapies in neurodegenerative disorders.

REFERENCES

Amor S, Puentes F, Baker D, van der Valk P 2010. Inflammation in neurodegenerative diseases *Immunology.* 129: 154-69.

Amor S, Smith PA, 't Hart LA and Baker D. 2005 Biozzi mice: Of mice and human neurological diseases. *J. Neuroimmunol.* 165: 1-10.

Amor S and 't Hart LA. 2003 Recombinant antibody fragments as autoantibody antagonists. *Expert opinions on Therapeutic Patents.* 13: 129-133.

Angelov DN, Waibel S, Guntinas-Lichius O, Lenzen M, Neiss WF, Tomov TL, Yoles E, Kipnis J, Schori H, Reuter A, Ludolph A, Schwartz M 2003. Therapeutic vaccine *Proc Natl Acad Sci U S A.* 100: 4790-5.

Baker D, Amor S. Quality control of experimental autoimmune encephalomyelitis *Mult. Scler.* 2010 16(9):1025-7.

Baptiste DC, Tighe A, Fehlings MG 2009. Spinal cord injury *Expert Opin. Investig. Drugs.* May;18(5):663-73.

Benner EJ, Mosley RL, Destache CJ, Lewis TB, Jackson-Lewis V, Gorantla S, Nemachek C, Green SR, Przedborski S, Gendelman HE 2004. Therapeutic immunization protects dopaminergic neurons in a mouse model of Parkinson's disease. *Proc Natl Acad Sci U S A.* 101: 9435-40.

Bielekova B, Becker BL 2010. Monoclonal antibodies in MS: mechanisms of action. *Neurology.*

Bittner S, Meuth SG, Göbel K, Melzer N, Herrmann AM, Simon OJ, Weishaupt A, Budde T, Bayliss DA, Bendszus M, Wiendl H 2009. TASK1 modulates inflammation and neurodegeneration in autoimmune inflammation of the central nervous system. *Brain.* 132(Pt 9): 2501-16.

Blesch A, Uy HS, Grill RJ, Cheng JG, Patterson PH, Tuszynski MH 1999. Leukemia inhibitory factor augments neurotrophin expression and corticospinal axon growth *J. Neurosci.* 19: 3556-66.

Block F, Pergande G, Schwarz M 1997. Flupirtine reduces functional deficits and neuronal damage after global ischemia *Brain Res.* 754(1-2): 279-84

Brinkmann V, Billich A, Baumruker T, Heining P, Schmouder R, Francis G, Aradhye S, Burtin P. Fingolimod (FTY720): discovery and development of an oral drug to treat multiple sclerosis. *Nat. Rev. Drug Discov.* 2010 Nov;9(11):883-97.

Brown RH Jr, Hauser SL, Harrington H, Weiner HL. Failure of immunosuppression *Arch. Neurol.* 1986 Apr;43(4):383-4.

Boutajangout A, Quartermain D, Sigurdsson EM. Immunotherapy targeting pathological tau prevents cognitive decline in a new tangle mouse model. *J. Neurosci.* 2010 Dec 8;30(49):16559-66.

Calvo A, Moglia C, Balma M, Chiò A. Involvement of immune response in the pathogenesis of amyotrophic lateral sclerosis: a therapeutic opportunity? *CNS* 2010 Jul;9(3):325-30.

Chang ZY, Chiang CH, Lu DW, Yeh MK. Erythropoiesis-stimulating protein delivery in providing erythropoiesis and neuroprotection *Expert Opin. Drug Deliv.* 2008 Dec;5(12):1313-21.

Chen Y, Meininger V, Guillemin GJ. Recent advances in the treatment of amyotrophic lateral sclerosis. Emphasis on kynurenine pathway inhibitors. *Cent. Nerv. Syst. Agents Med. Chem.* 2009 Mar;9(1):32-9.

Chen Y, Stankovic R, Cullen KM, Meininger V, Garner B, Coggan S, Grant R, Brew BJ, Guillemin GJ. The kynurenine pathway *Neurotox. Res.* 2010 Aug;18(2):132-42.

Citron M. Alzheimer's disease: strategies for disease modification. *Nat. Rev. Drug Discov.* 2010 May;9(5):387-98. .

Clifford DB, De Luca A, Simpson DM, Arendt G, Giovannoni G, Nath A. Natalizumab-associated progressive multifocal leukoencephalopathy *Lancet Neurol.* 2010 Apr;9(4):438-46.

Comi G. Treatment of multiple sclerosis *Neurol. Sci.* 2009 Oct;30 Suppl 2:S155-8.

Craggs L, Kalaria RN. Revisiting dietary antioxidants, neurodegeneration *Neuroreport.* 2010

Dittenhafer-Reed KE, Feldman JL, Denu JM. Catalysis and mechanistic insights into sirtuin activation. *Chembiochem.* 2011 Jan 24;12(2):281-9.

Drachman DB, Chaudhry V, Cornblath D, Kuncl RW, Pestronk A, Clawson L, Mellits ED, Quaskey S, Quinn T, Calkins A, et al. Trial of immunosuppression in amyotrophic lateral sclerosis using total lymphoid irradiation. *Ann. Neurol.* 1994 Feb;35(2):142-50.

Farrugia ME, Vincent A. Autoimmune mediated neuromuscular junction defects *Curr. Opin. Neurol.* 2010 Oct;23(5):489-95.

Fontoura P, Ho PP, DeVoss J, et al. Immunity to the extracellular domain of Nogo-A modulates experimental autoimmune encephalomyelitis. *J. Immunol.* 2004;173:6981Y92

Gunnarsson M, Malmeström C, Axelsson M, Sundström P, Dahle C, Vrethem M, Olsson T, Piehl F, Norgren N, Rosengren L, Svenningsson A, Lycke J. Axonal damage in relapsing multiple sclerosis *Ann. Neurol.* 2011 Jan;69(1):83-9.

Gold R, Kieseier BC Therapy of immune neuropathies with intravenous immunoglobulins *J. Neurol.* 2006 Sep;253 Suppl 5:V59-63.

Harbige LS, Layward L, Morris-Downes MM, Dumonde DC, Amor S. The protective effects of omega-6 fatty acids *Clin. Exp. Immunol.* 2000 Dec;122(3):445-52.

Harbige LS, Yeatman N, Amor S, Crawford MA. Prevention of experimental autoimmune encephalomyelitis *Br. J. Nutr.* 1995 Nov;74(5):701-15.

Harbige LS, Layward L, Morris M, Amor S. Protective mechanisms by omega-6 lipids *Biochem. Soc. Trans.* 1997 May;25(2):342S.

Harris and Amor S. Sweet and Sour - Oxidative and Carbonyl Stress in Neurological Disorders. *CNS Neurol. Disord. Drug Targets.* 2010.

Heijmans N, Smith PA, Morris-Downes MM, Pryce G, Baker D, Donaldson AV, 't Hart B, Amor S. Encephalitogenic and tolerogenic potential of altered peptide ligand *J. Neuroimmunol.* 2005 Oct;167(1-2):23-33.

Huang H, Benoist C, Mathis D. Rituximab specifically depletes short-lived autoreactive plasma cells in a mouse model of inflammatory arthritis. Proc *Natl. Acad. Sci. U. S. A.* 2010 Mar 9;107(10):4658-63. Epub 2010 Feb 22.

Kincses ZT, Toldi J, Vécsei L. Kynurenines, neurodegeneration and Alzheimer's disease. *J. Cell Mol. Med.* 2010.

Kumar S, Biancotti JC, Yamaguchi M, de Vellis J. Combination of growth *Neurochem. Res.* 2007 Apr-May;32(4-5):783-97.

Leist TP, Weissert R. Cladribine: mode of action and implications for treatment of multiple sclerosis. *Clin. Neuropharmacol.* 2011 Jan-Feb;34(1):28-35.

Lu L, Li F, Wang X Novel anti-inflammatory and neuroprotective agents for Parkinson's disease. *CNS* 2010 Apr;9(2):232-40.

Minagar A, Alexander JS, Sahraian MA, Zivadinov R. Alemtuzumab and multiple sclerosis *Expert Opin. Biol. Ther.* 2010 Mar;10(3):421-9.

Ortega-Gutiérrez S. Therapeutic perspectives of inhibitors of endocannabinoid degradation *Curr. Drug Targets CNS Neurol. Disord.* 2005 Dec;4(6):697-707.

Pelosof LC, Gerber DE.Paraneoplastic syndromes: an approach to diagnosis and treatment. *Mayo Clin. Proc.* 2010 Sep;85(9):838-54.

Pryce G, Ahmed Z, Hankey DJ, Jackson SJ, Croxford JL, Pocock JM, Ledent C, Petzold A, Thompson AJ, Giovannoni G, Cuzner ML, Baker D. Cannabinoids inhibit neurodegeneration *Brain.* 2003 Oct;126(Pt 10):2191-202.

Pryce G, O'Neill JK, Croxford JL, Amor S, Hankey DJ, East E, Giovannoni G, Baker D. Autoimmune tolerance eliminates relapses *J. Neuroimmunol.* 2005 Aug;165(1-2):41-52.

Racke MK, Lovett-Racke AE, Karandikar NJ.The mechanism of action of glatiramer acetate *Neurology.* 2010 Jan 5;74 Suppl 1:S25-30.

Rajda C, Bergquist J, Vécsei L. Kynurenines, redox disturbances and neurodegeneration in multiple sclerosis. *J. Neural Transm. Suppl.* 2007;(72):323-9.

Rossi S, Bernardi G, Centonze D. The endocannabinoid system in the inflammatory and neurodegenerative processes of multiple sclerosis *Exp. Neurol.* 2010 Jul;224(1):92-102.

Rupalla K, Cao W, Krieglstein J. Flupirtine protects neurons against excitotoxic or ischemic damage and inhibits the increase in cytosolic Ca2+ concentration. *Eur. J. Pharmacol.* 1995 Dec 29;294(2-3):469-73

Sättler MB, Williams SK, Neusch C, Otto M, Pehlke JR, Bähr M, Diem R. Flupirtine as neuroprotective add-on therapy in autoimmune optic neuritis. *Am. J. Pathol.* 2008 Nov;173(5):1496-507. Epub 2008 Oct 2.

Simonen M, Pedersen V, Weinmann O, et al. Systemic deletion of the myelin-associated outgrowth inhibitor Nogo-A improves regenerative and plastic responses after spinal cord injury. *Neuron.* 2003;38:201Y11

Shi R, Sun W. Potassium channel blockers as an effective treatment to restore impulse conduction in injured axons. *Neurosci. Bull.* 2011 Feb;27(1):36-44.

Smith PA, Morris-Downes M, Heijmans N, Pryce G, Arter E, O'Neill JK, 't Hart B, Baker D, Amor S. Epitope spread is not critical for the relapse and progression of MOG *J. Neuroimmunol.* 2005 Jul;164(1-2):76-84.

Stone TW. Inhibitors of the kynurenine pathway *Eur. J. Med. Chem.* 2000 Feb;35(2):179-86. Review.

Thevandavakkam MA, Schwarcz R, Muchowski PJ, Giorgini F. Targeting kynurenine 3-monooxygenase (KMO): implications for therapy in Huntington's disease. *CNS* 2010 Dec;9(6):791-800.

van Noort JM, Bsibsi M, Gerritsen WH, van der Valk P, Bajramovic JJ, Steinman L, Amor S. Alphab-crystallin is a target *J. Neuropathol. Exp. Neurol.* 2010 Jul;69(7):694-703.

van der Valk P, Amor S. Preactive lesions *Curr. Opin. Neurol.* 2009 Jun;22(3):207-13. Review.

Vesterinen HM, Sena ES, ffrench-Constant C, Williams A, Chandran S, Macleod MR. Improving the translational hit of experimental treatments in multiple sclerosis. *Mult. Scler.* 2010 Sep;16(9):1044-55.

INDEX

J

K

L

M

N

O